BEHIND THE SMILE

THE UNSEEN SIGNS OF EMOTIONAL ABUSE

How to Recognize, Support, and Prevent Controlling
Relationships with Those You Love

BY TIFFINY NEWTON

Published by 1BrickPublishing
Printed in the United States
Copyright © 2024 by Tiffiny Newton
ISBN 978-1949303421

DEDICATION

To those who are enduring the silent battles and wearing
unseen scars,

and to the loved ones who, through patience and
understanding,

help us find our way back to ourselves.

May this book serve as a light for those navigating the shadows,

a reminder to release shame and guilt, and to recognize that we
are brave warriors. Healing, courage, and self-worth are always
within reach.

For my family, friends, and every survivor—your strength
inspires this work.

DEDICATION REQUEST

Please share this book with anyone you feel could benefit from its insights, support, and guidance in recognizing, preventing, and healing from emotional abuse. May it serve as a source of strength, awareness, and empowerment for all who seek a path to healthier, safer relationships.

Table of Contents

INTRODUCTION

WHY WE CAN'T IGNORE EMOTIONAL AND PSYCHOLOGICAL ABUSE

When people think of abuse, they often picture physical violence—bruises, broken bones, or visible scars. But the scars left by emotional and psychological abuse run just as deep, if not deeper, and they are often hidden in plain sight. I know this all too well because I lived through it. For years, I was trapped in a relationship that slowly eroded my confidence, my identity, and my sense of self-worth. It wasn't until I was deep in the abyss of manipulation, coercion, surveillance, and control that I realized what was happening to me—and by then, I felt like I was losing my mind.

My story is not unique. Like many survivors of emotional and psychological abuse, I didn't see the warning signs. It started so subtly that I had no reason to suspect anything was wrong. After all, the person I thought I loved seemed caring, attentive, and invested in our relationship. He was charming, generous, and protective. But over time, the cracks in that perfect facade began to show.

It began with comments that seemed insignificant at the time. He would tell me he didn't like how my friends acted or how they were interfering in my time with him. He'd say, "I'm just looking out for you," and I believed him. Who wouldn't want a partner who cared so much? But soon, those little comments turned into demands: "I don't want you hanging out with them anymore." "How could you be friends with someone who is so disrespectful?" Slowly, I started pulling away from the people who cared about me.

Isolation is a key tactic in emotional and psychological abuse, and it's so subtle that you often don't realize it's happening until it's too late. By the time I noticed how alone I had become, I was already deep in the relationship, and I had convinced myself that my partner was the only one who truly understood me.

The love bombing, the intense attention, the constant contact—it all felt so overwhelming and, at times, intoxicating. But it was also suffocating. There was no space for me to be my own person. If I wasn't constantly available, constantly answering his calls or texts, he would get upset. He would accuse me of not caring, of not prioritizing our relationship. And every time I questioned whether his behavior was normal, he would turn it around on me: "I'm just looking out for us. Don't you want this to work?"

It wasn't until the manipulation escalated that I began to see the situation for what it was. He monitored my social media, made cruel comments about how I dressed, and controlled where I went and who I saw. He used my own insecurities against me, convincing me that I wasn't good enough and that I was lucky to have him. And all the while, he maintained that this was love—that he was protecting me from a world that didn't understand me the way he did.

By the time I realized the full extent of his control, I had lost so much of myself. I had become someone I didn't recognize—constantly walking on eggshells, afraid to say or do the wrong thing, and feeling like it was all my fault. What's worse is that I had internalized his narrative about who I was, and I felt powerless to escape.

It took years of rebuilding my self-worth and unraveling the emotional and psychological damage he had caused for me to finally break free. I am sharing my story not to evoke pity, but to show just how insidious emotional and psychological abuse can be. It can happen to anyone—no matter how strong, independent, or confident you are. The tactics used by emotional abusers are designed to break down even the most resilient person, and they work slowly, almost imperceptibly, until you find yourself trapped in a cycle of control and manipulation.

But there is hope. I survived, and I've made it my mission to help others recognize the signs of emotional and psychological abuse before it's too late. My story is not just a cautionary tale—it's a call to action. Emotional and psychological abuse can be prevented, but only if we are equipped to recognize it for what it is.

Emotional and psychological abuse is one of the most misunderstood and dismissed forms of abuse. Because it doesn't leave visible scars, it's easy to ignore or overlook. But make no mistake—emotional and psychological abuse is just as damaging, and sometimes even more so, than physical violence. It chips away at a person's self-esteem, their sense of identity, and their ability to trust themselves and others.

The damage caused by emotional and psychological abuse can last long after the relationship ends. Survivors are left with deep psychological wounds that can take years to heal. The constant manipulation, gaslighting, and control leave victims doubting their own perceptions and questioning their reality. It's not uncommon for survivors to feel as though they've lost themselves entirely.

What makes emotional and psychological abuse so dangerous is that it's often difficult to recognize. It's not as obvious as a slap or a punch. Instead, it manifests through words, actions, and behaviors that, on the surface, may seem benign or even loving. The abuser may seem caring, attentive, and protective. They may present themselves as the perfect partner—someone who is always there for you, always looking out for you. But behind that facade is a need for control, a desire to dominate and manipulate.

Emotional abusers use a variety of tactics to achieve control. They may isolate their partner from friends and family, making them feel as though they have no one to turn to. They may use gaslighting to make their partner doubt their own memories and perceptions. They may be overly critical, constantly putting their partner down or making them feel inadequate. And they often use an overwhelming display of affection and attention—called love bombing—to keep their partner hooked, even as the abuse escalates.

The insidious nature of emotional and psychological abuse means that many victims don't even realize they're being abused. They may feel that something is wrong in their relationship, but they can't quite put their finger on it. They may believe that their partner's behavior is normal, or that they're overreacting. And because emotional abusers often present themselves as charming and loving to the outside world, friends and family may not see the abuse either.

This is why emotional and psychological abuse can go on for so long—years, even decades—without being addressed. Victims are left to suffer in silence, often believing that they are the problem, that they can fix the situation by changing their behavior, and that they are unworthy of love or respect. The long-term effects of this kind of abuse can be devastating, leading to anxiety, depression, and even post-traumatic stress disorder (PTSD) and C-PTSD (complex PTSD).

This book is important because it shines a light on the unseen danger of emotional and psychological manipulation. It gives voice to those who have suffered in silence, and it provides the tools necessary to recognize abuse for what it is—a form of control and domination that strips away a person's autonomy and self-worth.

In addition to the emotional and psychological scars, coercive control leaves deep imprints on the lives of survivors. It operates silently, slipping into daily routines and relationships, sometimes so subtly that even the victim may not realize it's happening until they are deeply entrenched in a web of control. My personal experience taught me that coercive control doesn't just involve physical violence—it permeates every aspect of life, from finances to friendships, and even our own sense of self-worth.

For me, the realization came too late. I was manipulated into cutting off long-standing friendships simply because my abuser didn't "approve" of them. He framed it as concern for my well-being, saying these people were distractions or didn't have my best interests at heart. Slowly, I found myself isolated from the people I had known for years, trapped in a relationship where every email, every text, and every social media message was monitored and controlled. He even went so far as to send demeaning messages from my accounts to people I cared about, ruining relationships and further tightening his control over my life.

Whether you are a friend, family member, or partner of someone you suspect is in an emotionally and psychologically abusive relationship, this book will help you understand the warning signs and how to provide the support they need. If you are someone who has experienced emotional or psychological abuse, this book will offer you validation, guidance, and hope for healing.

The primary goal of this book is to educate loved ones—friends, family members, and partners—on how to recognize the signs of emotional and psychological abuse and how to provide meaningful support to those who are trapped in abusive relationships. Emotional and psychological abuse thrives in secrecy and isolation, and the best way to combat it is through awareness and understanding.

Throughout this book, you will learn how emotional and psychological abusers operate, the tactics they use to control and manipulate, and the red flags to watch for. But this book is not just about recognizing abuse—it's also about taking action. You'll learn how to approach a loved one who may be in an abusive relationship, how to offer support without judgment, and how to help them regain their sense of self-worth and autonomy.

One of the most important aspects of supporting someone in an emotionally and psychologically abusive relationship is understanding that leaving is not always easy. Abusers are often skilled at making their victims feel dependent on them, and the psychological toll of the abuse can make it difficult for the victim to see a way out. As a loved one, your role is to be a source of strength and support, offering compassion and patience as the victim navigates their journey toward healing.

This book also emphasizes the importance of prevention. By educating young people about the signs of emotional manipulation and teaching them to value their self-worth, we can help prevent them from entering into abusive relationships in the first place. We need to have these conversations early, before the damage is done.

Ultimately, this book is a call to action. Emotional and psychological abuse is a pervasive and damaging problem, but it doesn't have to continue unchecked. By recognizing the signs and taking steps to intervene, we can help those we love break free from the cycle of abuse and reclaim their lives.

Let this book be your guide in navigating the complex and often hidden world of emotional and psychological abuse. Together, we can create a future where no one has to suffer in silence.

CHAPTER 1

UNDERSTANDING EMOTIONAL AND PSYCHOLOGICAL ABUSE

E motional and psychological abuse can be difficult to spot, especially in the early stages of a relationship. Use this quick reference guide to identify red flags and patterns that may indicate emotional abuse. These signs may appear in romantic relationships, friendships, family relationships, or even workplace dynamics.

When we think of abuse, what typically comes to mind? For many of us, it's physical violence—visible bruises, broken bones, or someone being physically hurt. But here's the thing: not all abuse leaves marks you can see. Emotional and psychological abuse can be just as damaging, if not more so, and the scars it leaves are often invisible. These are the kinds of scars that run deep, lingering in your mind and heart long after the abuse has ended.

I know this all too well because I've lived it.

Emotional abuse is a form of manipulation aimed at controlling how someone feels. It might involve making someone question their worth, isolating them from loved ones, or constantly criticizing them. **Psychological abuse**, on the other hand, digs deeper—it targets the way someone thinks, the decisions they make, and their sense of reality. It's about controlling a person's thoughts and behaviors, often through intimidation, threats, and constant surveillance. It's subtle but powerful.

Coercive control, while less visible than physical violence, is often more insidious and far-reaching. It manifests in countless ways, gradually eroding the autonomy and self-worth of the victim. Statistics show that 99% of abusive relationships consist of financial abuse. One of the most profound examples in my life was the complete control over my finances. I was made to feel guilty about every financial decision, coerced into justifying every expenditure—even though the money was mine. Eventually, I was manipulated out of $40,000 from my retirement account, a decision that left me financially devastated and emotionally crushed. This financial exploitation is a common yet less-discussed tactic used by abusers to maintain control.

But coercive control doesn't stop at money. I remember the day that my abuser didn't like something he discovered on my phone; he then decided to bend it to the point where it was unusable. The violence was not just physical but symbolic; it was a reminder that everything in my life, down to my communication with the outside world, was under his control. He had installed cameras in our home, monitoring my every move, stripping away any sense of privacy or personal autonomy. This wasn't just about control; it was about domination.

These experiences taught me that emotional abuse is not just about cruel words or manipulative behaviors—it's about stripping someone of their independence, their privacy, and their ability to trust themselves. And this is why recognizing emotional abuse is so crucial: the sooner we see it, the sooner we can stop it.

For years, I was in a relationship that chipped away at who I was—slowly, subtly, and in ways I didn't even realize at first. It didn't start with shouting or violence; in fact, it started with what felt like love. My partner showered me with attention and affection. I felt like the most important person in the world, but over time, that attention turned into control, and that affection became a weapon used against me.

In my case, the abuse crept up on me. My partner started by saying things like, "I just want what's best for us," or "It's us against the world." It seemed caring at first, like he was protecting me. But eventually, those comments turned into, "Are they more important to you than I am?," or "You're wearing that? You're trying to impress someone else?"

It felt like love at first. I thought, "Wow, this person really cares about me." But what I didn't realize at the time was that this "care" was a way to isolate me, to make me depend on him entirely. And slowly, I was isolated from my friends and started pulling away from my family.

The Spectrum of Abuse

Abuse isn't always loud or obvious. Sometimes it's quiet, sneaky, and disguised as love or concern. There's a wide spectrum when it comes to abuse, and emotional and psychological abuse sit at the quieter end of that spectrum, often making it harder to spot.

In my experience, **emotional abuse** looked like this:

- **Gaslighting**: He would make me doubt my own memories and feelings. I remember telling him something he'd said hurt me, and his response was, "You're being too sensitive. I never said that." Over time, I started questioning whether my feelings were valid at all.
- **Constant criticism**: Nothing I did was ever right. Whether it was how I dressed, who I talked to, or the decisions I made, there was always something wrong in his eyes. He would say things like, "You really think

that's what you should wear today?" or "I don't know why you don't stick up for me."

- **Isolation**: This is one of the biggest red flags I missed early on. At first, it was just suggestions—"Let's go workout at the gym together." Then it became stronger: "I don't want you going to the gym without me." Before I knew it, I was completely cut off from the people who cared about me and activities I loved.

On the other side, **psychological abuse** went even deeper:

- **Intimidation and control**: He kept tabs on everything I did—who I talked to, where I went, even how I dressed. I started feeling like I had to explain my every move, constantly afraid of upsetting him.

- **Surveillance**: He monitored my social media, went through my phone, tracked my location, and even installed cameras in our condo to keep an eye on me. It wasn't just about controlling what I did; it was about controlling what I thought, who I could trust, and how much freedom I was allowed.

- **Threats**: While there were no overt threats of violence, the underlying message was clear: "If you don't do things my way, there will be consequences." Those consequences might be emotional and physical withdrawal, coldness, or endless arguments. But the fear was always there.

Coercive control encapsulates many of these abusive behaviors. It's a pattern of manipulation designed to undermine a person's autonomy and sense of self. Survivors may find themselves isolated from friends and family, compelled into compliance, and stripped of their personal agency.

Recognizing coercive control is crucial for understanding the broader landscape of emotional abuse. Tactics such as constant monitoring, dictating personal choices, and instilling fear through intimidation thrive on confusion and secrecy. This makes it essential for survivors and their allies to identify and confront these harmful dynamics.

What's particularly unsettling about emotional and psychological abuse is that they often masquerade as love, care, or protection. This deceptive disguise makes it easy to fall into the trap without even realizing it, blurring the lines between genuine affection and controlling behavior.

Why It's So Hard to See Emotional and Psychological Abuse

It's so easy to look back and see things clearly. But when you're living in an emotionally or psychologically abusive relationship, it's much harder to recognize the signs. Abusers are often charming, attentive, and caring at first. It's part of the grooming process. They reel you in with love and affection, making you feel like you've found the perfect partner. But little by little, that affection turns into control.

I didn't wake up one day and suddenly find myself isolated and scared. It happened gradually. At first, I was flattered by his attention. He was always checking in, wanting to know how my day was going, where I was and who I was with. It felt like love, like he was truly interested in me. But over time, I realized it wasn't about love at all—it was about control.

One of the hardest parts about emotional and psychological abuse is that it doesn't leave physical marks. There are no bruises or scars to point to and say, "See, this is what's happening to me." Instead, the damage is internal. It's the constant self-doubt, the fear of making the wrong move, and the gradual erosion of your confidence and identity.

For me, it took years to really recognize what was happening. By the time I realized the full extent of his control, I had lost so much of myself. I didn't trust my own judgment. I couldn't make decisions without second-guessing myself, I thought I was losing my mind. And I felt like I had nowhere to turn because I had already distanced myself from the people who could help.

That's what makes emotional and psychological abuse so dangerous—it's invisible. It works its way into your mind and heart, making you question everything, until you feel like there's no way out.

The Dismissal of Emotional and Psychological Abuse

It's frustrating how often emotional and psychological abuse are dismissed or downplayed. People tend to think that unless you're being hit or physically hurt, it's not "real" abuse. But that mindset couldn't be further from the truth. Emotional scars can last just as long, if not longer, than physical ones.

I can't count how many times I was told, "Just get over it" or "You're overreacting" or "That didn't happen." It's common for people on the outside to think that because there are no visible injuries, it's not that bad. But what they don't see are the nights spent crying because you don't know why you feel so broken. They don't see the constant anxiety or the way you start to lose your sense of who you are.

Society has a lot of misconceptions about abuse. We're taught to believe that relationships are supposed to be hard, that love involves sacrifice. But there's a line between compromise and control, and emotional abusers are experts at making you believe their behavior is just part of that "sacrifice." They'll tell you they're only trying to protect you, that they're just looking out for your best interests. And because there are no physical marks, it's easy to start believing them.

The truth is, abuse is abuse—whether it leaves physical scars or not. We need to start recognizing that emotional and psychological abuse are just as harmful, if not more so, because of how deeply they affect a person's mental and emotional well-being.

The Long-Term Impact of Emotional and Psychological Abuse

The effects of emotional and psychological abuse don't end when the relationship does. In fact, the hardest part comes after you leave—when you're left to pick up the pieces of who you used to be.

For me, leaving wasn't the end of the abuse—it was the beginning of the healing process. I had to relearn how to trust myself, how to make decisions without second-guessing everything. I had to rebuild my confidence from the ground up because for so long, I had been told that I wasn't good enough, smart enough, or worthy of love.

Emotional and psychological abuse leaves you with deep emotional scars—scars that can lead to anxiety, depression, PTSD and even C-PTSD. It can take years to heal, and even then, the effects may linger.

The hardest part is learning to trust again. After living in a constant state of fear and control, opening myself up to new relationships felt impossible. I questioned everyone's motives, wondering if they, too, would try to control me. It took time, therapy, and a lot of self-reflection to rebuild my sense of self and my ability to trust others.

The Importance of Recognizing the Signs

The sooner emotional and psychological abuse is recognized, the easier it is to stop the cycle. For those of us on the outside—friends, family, and loved ones—it's crucial to pay attention to the signs. In many cases, the victim won't even realize what's happening to them, or they'll feel too ashamed or scared to talk about it.

Some signs to watch for include:

- **Behavioral changes**: Has your loved one become more withdrawn, anxious, or isolated?
- **Over-dependence on their partner**: Do they seem overly reliant on their partner's approval or afraid to make decisions without consulting them first?
- **Unexplained Emotional Distress:** Are they frequently upset or anxious but unable to explain why?
- **Loss of interest:** Have they stopped engaging in activities they once enjoyed or distanced themselves from friends and family?
- **Self-doubt and criticism:** Do they often express feelings of worthlessness or inadequacy, or do they seem to be overly critical of themselves?

- **Walking on eggshells**: Does it seem like they're constantly afraid of saying or doing the wrong thing?

As someone who has been there, I can tell you that recognizing these signs and offering support can make all the difference. It's not always easy, but paying close attention and being present for your loved ones can help them break free from the cycle of abuse before it's too late.

The Nature of Emotional and Psychological Abuse

One of the most challenging aspects of emotional and psychological abuse is that it's often invisible—not just to the people around you, but sometimes even to the victim themselves. When I was going through it, I didn't think of myself as someone who was being abused. The word "abuse" felt too extreme for what I thought was just a difficult relationship.

But that's the trick. Emotional and psychological abuse don't announce themselves with the same clarity as physical abuse. It starts small—so small that you might not even notice it at first. It could be a few well-placed comments, like humiliation disguised as humor, can make you doubt yourself. Your partner's seeming "concern" about your whereabouts can feel like love, but it quickly becomes suffocating.

The emotional abuse I experienced was not my abuser yelling at me every day. It began as a quiet erosion of who I was. Every little criticism, every small dig at my choices, every moment I was made to feel "less than" added up. And the worst part? The more it happened, the more I believed it. I started to think, "Maybe I'm too sensitive. Maybe I am making a big deal out of nothing."

That's the nature of emotional and psychological abuse—it makes you doubt yourself. It convinces you that you are the problem.

In my experience, the control came in waves. There would be good days when everything felt fine, maybe even great, but those days were just enough to make me overlook the bad ones. It's a cycle that keeps you hanging on, hoping things will improve, convincing yourself that maybe it's just a rough patch. And every time you convince yourself that the relationship is worth saving, the abuse digs in a little deeper.

Why Emotional and Psychological Abuse Are Often Dismissed

People often ask why victims of emotional and psychological abuse don't just leave. "If it's that bad, why stay?" they ask. But here's the thing—it's not always that easy.

Part of the difficulty in recognizing emotional and psychological abuse is that it doesn't fit the stereotypical image of abuse. There are no visible marks or broken bones. Instead, there are whispered insults, constant criticism, and a feeling that you're losing control over your life—but those experiences are harder to prove. Because there's nothing tangible to show, people tend to dismiss it. Sometimes you just feel like you are losing your mind, so maybe they are right.

I can't count how many times I heard things like, "You guys have such a great relationship" or "What a fun trip you went on." People around me didn't see the full picture because emotional abuse thrives in secrecy. And what is shared publicly - especially on social media - is a front, a controlled view into how wonderful your lives are together. You don't walk around telling people how controlled you feel. In fact, many victims, including myself, feel ashamed or embarrassed to admit they are being manipulated.

Then there's society's misconceptions. We're conditioned to believe that relationships are supposed to be hard, that love requires sacrifice. So when you find yourself in a controlling or manipulative situation, it's easy to brush it off as "normal relationship problems." After all, no relationship is perfect, right? But we must draw the line.

It's not just about the difficult moments that come with any relationship; it's about harmful patterns of behavior that are designed to tear you down. Abusers disguise their actions as love or care, saying things like, "I'm only doing this because I care about you," or "I just want what's best for you." And after hearing those words over and over, you start to believe them.

The Long-Term Impact of Emotional and Psychological Abuse

The effects of emotional and psychological abuse don't just vanish once the relationship ends. For me, the hardest part wasn't walking away, it was trying to rebuild my life after. It's like standing in the middle of a wreckage, unsure where to start.

When your sense of self has been systematically torn apart, it can take a long time to feel like "you" again. I spent years doubting every decision I made, questioning my judgment, and trying to regain the lost confidence. Even in new relationships, the fear lingered. I was constantly waiting for the other shoe to drop, expecting every new person I met to turn into my abuser.

One of the worst effects of emotional abuse is how it warps your sense of reality. Gaslighting, in particular, made me question my own memories and perception of events. There were times when I couldn't even trust my own thoughts because I had been told for so long that I was wrong, that I was overreacting, or that something I saw wasn't true. That doubt doesn't just disappear; it lingers, making it difficult to trust others—and even more difficult to trust yourself.

Then there's the anxiety. Emotional abuse leaves you in a constant state of alertness. Even after the abuse ends, your mind is still on edge, still waiting for the next emotional blow. I found myself overanalyzing conversations, interactions, wondering if I had said or done something wrong, or if I had somehow disappointed him.

For many survivors of emotional and psychological abuse, recovery is a long road. It's not just about leaving the relationship; it's about reclaiming and rebuilding who you are. That journey takes time, patience, and a lot of self-compassion.

The Importance of Recognizing the Signs

One of the hardest parts about emotional and psychological abuse is that it often flies under the radar. For the victim, it's difficult to see when you're in it. And for loved ones on the outside, the signs can be even harder to spot. That's why recognizing the red flags is so important.

I didn't realize how much I had changed until it was almost too late. I stopped hanging out with my friends, stopped communicating with my family as much, and my world revolved entirely around him—his approval, his needs, his happiness. I became quieter, more anxious, always on edge.

Looking back, the signs were so clear. I felt like I had to walk on eggshells around him, stopped making decisions for myself, and constantly apologized–even when I hadn't done anything wrong. But I was in so deep that I couldn't see the truth.

For friends and family, it's vital to pay attention to these changes. If someone you love suddenly becomes withdrawn or overly dependent on their partner, it might be time to ask some tough questions. It's not easy to intervene, but sometimes it's necessary.

Signs to look out for:

- **Isolation**: Have they cut off contact with friends and family? Are they spending all their time with their partner, neglecting their own life?
- **Walking on eggshells**: Do they seem nervous or afraid to speak their mind? Are they constantly apologizing, even for things that aren't their fault?
- **Over-dependence on their partner**: Are they afraid to make decisions without their partner's input? Do they overtly prioritize their partner's opinions, even on trivial matters?

Recognizing these signs and offering support can make all the difference. Sometimes, all it takes is someone noticing that something is wrong to start the process of breaking free.

Understanding the Cycles of Abuse

To truly grasp the complexities of emotional and psychological abuse, it's crucial to understand the cycles that often define these destructive relationships. The cycle of abuse consists of four distinct phases: tension-building, incident, reconciliation, and calm. Recognizing these cycles can help survivors and their supporters understand the patterns at play and the reasons behind them.

Tension-Building Phase: This phase is marked by increasing stress and strain in the relationship. The abuser may become increasingly irritable, critical, or controlling, leading to an environment of fear and anxiety for the victim. The victim may feel like they are walking on eggshells, constantly trying to appease the abuser to avoid conflict. This phase can last days, weeks, or even longer, creating a sense of impending doom.

Incident Phase: This is the point where the abuse occurs. It may manifest as verbal outbursts, emotional manipulation, or other forms of coercive control. The intensity of the incident can vary, but the impact on the victim is often profound and damaging. During this phase, the abuser may use tactics like gaslighting, which can leave the victim questioning their reality and feeling isolated.

Reconciliation Phase: After the incident, many abusers engage in a period of "honeymooning." They may apologize profusely, express regret, and promise to change. This can create confusion for the victim, as the abuser's charm and remorse may lead them to believe that the relationship can return to normal. Victims may feel a glimmer of hope, wanting to believe that the abuser can change.

Calm Phase: This phase involves a temporary sense of peace. The abuser may seem loving and attentive, and the victim might feel relieved. However, this calm is often deceptive, as it sets the stage for the tension-building phase to begin again. Over time, the calm phase may shorten, and the tension may escalate more quickly, making it harder for victims to escape the cycle.

Understanding these cycles is essential for both survivors and their supporters. It sheds light on why leaving an abusive relationship can be so difficult, as the cycle creates a confusing blend of hope, fear, and control. Many victims may feel trapped, believing that they are responsible for the abuser's behavior or that the reconciliation phase signifies real change.

By recognizing these patterns, you can empower yourself and others to identify the signs of emotional abuse and take proactive steps toward healing and liberation. Awareness is the first step in breaking the cycle and creating a future free from manipulation and control.

Emotional and psychological abuse are powerful, often invisible forces that can consume a person without them even realizing it. It's subtle, insidious, and incredibly damaging. But it doesn't have to be a life sentence. By recognizing the signs, speaking up, and offering support, we can help break the cycle of abuse.

For anyone who finds themselves in an emotionally or psychologically abusive relationship, know this: you are not alone, and you are not powerless. The first step toward healing is recognizing that something is wrong. And once you take that step, there is a path to recovery. Healing is possible. Recovery is real.

For loved ones, the best thing you can do is be there. Listen. Support. Help your friend or family member find their way back to themselves. Emotional and psychological abuse thrive in isolation, but with love and support, victims can—and do—find their way out.

CHAPTER 2

RECOGNIZING THE UNSEEN SIGNS

One of the hardest parts about emotional and psychological abuse is how difficult it can be to see, even when it's happening right in front of you. Most of us have an idea of what abuse looks like—bruises, shouting, fear—but emotional and psychological abuse don't always come with such clear markers. In fact, they often show up dressed as something else, something that can look like love or concern at first.

I remember thinking, "This is just how relationships are supposed to be, right? Love is intense. It's supposed to be all-consuming." And that's how it started—with intensity. I was swept up in the attention, the affection, the constant texts and calls. At the time, it felt flattering, like I was the center of his world. But looking back, I see now that what I thought was love was really the beginning of control.

That's the insidious nature of emotional and psychological abuse—it starts small. In the beginning, it doesn't feel like abuse. In fact, it often feels like love. But over time, the control tightens, and what was once flattering becomes suffocating.

The Grooming Process: From Love Bombing to Control

Abusers rarely start by showing their true colors. They don't begin by isolating you or controlling your every move. Instead, they start with what we call **love bombing**—an overwhelming display of affection, attention, and validation. It's intoxicating, pulling you in quickly.

The **grooming process** happens in stages. First, the abuser makes you feel special, loved, and adored. They give you everything you want—attention, time, affection. It feels like a whirlwind romance, and you become emotionally invested very quickly. They are the one "you've been searching for". But then, once they've hooked you, things start to change. Slowly, almost invisibly, they begin to exert control.

For me, it started with little things. He would say, "I just want to spend more time with you," which sounded sweet at first. But soon, it became, "Why are you spending time on your phone? You should only be using social media to post about how great our relationship is." And eventually, it turned into, "I don't want you being friends with them anymore. They are destructive to our relationship." And "Why haven't you posted anything about me or us on your Facebook in a while?"

He didn't start by making demands. He started by making me feel like I was the most important person in his life. When the demands came, they seemed justified. I didn't want to lose that feeling of being loved so intensely, so I started to give in. I stopped messaging my friends. I stopped taking time for myself. I started giving more and more of myself until I didn't recognize who I was anymore.

That's how **love bombing** turns into control. It's not an abrupt change; it's gradual, subtle, and sly. By the time I realized what was happening, I was already deep into the relationship, and pulling away felt impossible.

Early Warning Signs of Emotional and Psychological Abuse

Looking back, I can see the signs that were there from the very beginning. They were small—so small that I barely noticed them at the time. But those early warning signs were the cracks that eventually grew into the full-blown abuse I would later experience.

Here are some of the early warning signs I wish I'd recognized sooner:

1. **Constant contact**: At first, it felt flattering that he wanted to text and call all the time. I thought, "Wow, he must really like me." But over time, I realized that it wasn't about love—it was about keeping tabs on me. If I didn't respond right away, he would get upset, asking why I wasn't answering and who I was with.

2. **Isolation**: This started so subtly that I didn't even notice it as isolation at first. He would say things like, "I don't think your friends care about you as much as I do," or "I hired someone to do your hair here at the house." Slowly, he distanced me from the people who had always been there for me because I believed him when he said that he was the only one who truly understood me.

3. **Criticism disguised as concern**: He would often say things like, "I just want to help you be your best self," which sounds nice, right? But then he would criticize everything from how I dressed to how I handled situations at work. He made me feel like I couldn't do anything right without his input.

These behaviors might seem insignificant at first, but over time, they started to add up. They chipped away at my sense of self, making me more dependent on my abuser for validation and approval. By the time the more overt forms of control set in,

I was already emotionally hooked, making it harder to see the abuse for what it is. He had already changed my reality.

How Emotional Abuse Slowly Erodes Self-Worth and Independence

One of the most painful things about emotional abuse is how it sneaks up on you. It doesn't happen all at once. It unfolds gradually, over time, in ways that are easy to dismiss or explain away. You start to lose pieces of yourself without even realizing it.

For me, the loss of independence happened so gradually that by the time I noticed it, I had already given so much of myself away. It started with small compromises—canceling plans with friends because he wanted to spend time together, changing the way I dressed because he didn't like certain outfits, avoiding certain topics because I knew they would lead to a fight. But over time, those small compromises turned into bigger ones.

I used to be independent, confident, and self-assured. But little by little, I started to question myself. Every decision I made seemed to require his approval. If he didn't like something I said or did, I found myself apologizing, even when I hadn't done anything wrong. I began to believe that maybe I wasn't good enough on my own, that I needed his guidance and input to make the right choices.

Emotional abuse erodes your sense of self-worth in such a subtle way that you don't even realize it's happening. You start to believe the lies you're being told, that you're not capable, that you're not smart enough, or that you're too emotional. And before you know it, you're completely dependent on the person who is causing the damage.

My independence didn't disappear overnight. It was taken from me piece by piece, and by the time I realized what had happened, I felt trapped. The more control he took, the less I believed I could survive without him.

Missed Red Flags

Early warning signs in relationships are often dismissed as minor issues or quirks, but when they accumulate, they form a clear pattern of abuse. In my case, it began with seemingly innocuous comments: subtle critiques of my appearance for work, or casual suggestions about who I should or shouldn't spend time with. What felt like minor concerns eventually escalated into something far more dangerous.

One of the first signs of control came through my communication. He forced me to delete an old email account simply because it contained correspondence from previous relationships, even though those conversations had ended years ago. I was also made to discard certain books he disapproved of, like my collection of classic love poems. Over time, his paranoia about my connections with others became all-encompassing, narrowing my social world until there was no one left but him.

His control extended to every aspect of my daily life. When I wanted to get my hair done, instead of allowing me to go to a salon of my choosing, he arranged for a stylist to come to the house—where he could keep an eye on me and listen to my conversations. It wasn't about convenience; it was about asserting dominance over my autonomy.

Perhaps the most unsettling development was his installation of surveillance cameras throughout our home. What began as a "nanny cam for security" soon turned into multiple cameras placed in the hallway, living room, and even the bedroom. He needed to monitor my every move, and if anything disrupted this system—like the cameras going offline—he would immediately call me, no matter the hour, to fix it. These behaviors were subtle at first, but they painted a clear picture of escalating control and manipulation.

Looking back, I see the signs that I missed. At the time, I convinced myself he was simply protective, that his criticism was meant to help me. But now I understand that what I dismissed as care were actually early indicators of deeper abuse.

The need for control didn't present itself through grand gestures. It started small—like telling me what to wear or dictating who I could talk to. Initially, it felt like he was just offering advice, but over time, I realized that his "opinions" were non-negotiable rules. If I didn't comply, there were consequences—silent treatment, aggressive behavior, or emotional manipulation that left me feeling guilty for not meeting his expectations.

Another early sign of his controlling nature was his insistence on being involved in every facet of my life. At first, I thought it was sweet that he wanted to spend so much time with me, but soon, it became suffocating. My world began to shrink, and I wasn't allowed to have any part of my life that didn't include him. Social engagements with friends or family were met with guilt trips or complaints about how I wasn't prioritizing our relationship. Gradually, I pulled away from the people who cared about me, not even realizing that I was isolating myself under his influence.

What impacted me the most was how he made me feel about myself. Slowly but surely, I began to question my worth. His constant criticism, disguised as concern, made me second-guess every decision I made. Over time, I started to believe that I needed him to be the best version of myself. His manipulations chipped away at my confidence until I no longer trusted my own judgment.

The erosion of my self-worth wasn't an immediate or dramatic shift—it was a gradual process. One day, I was simply picking out an outfit for work, and he told me I didn't look professional enough. "You need to cover up more and wear flats," he said. Wanting to please him, I changed. But it didn't stop there. Soon, I found myself dressing to meet his preferences, whether we were going out or staying in. It soon became a requirement to dress how he wanted in order to keep him in a pleasant mood. I didn't even notice how much of myself I was giving up, little by little.

This control seeped into every part of my life. My career decisions, how I interacted with anyone, even the food I ate—all revolved around his desires. He made me feel like his opinions were superior, and if I ever disagreed or pushed back, I was made to feel like I was the one being unreasonable.

Emotional abuse works this way—it makes you doubt yourself at every turn. You start to believe that maybe you are too emotional, or overreacting, or that you really do need their guidance to make the right choices. And as the doubts creep in, your self-esteem slowly crumbles.

Before I knew it, I wasn't just dressing to please him—I was living to please him. Every decision, every step I took was calculated to avoid his disapproval. My own desires, goals, and happiness took a backseat as my life became an extension of his wants. I lost sight of who I was.

In hindsight, I can see all the signs that I missed. But at the time, they didn't feel like warning signs. They felt like the normal compromises people make in relationships when they love someone. What I didn't realize then is that there's a stark difference between healthy compromise and giving up pieces of yourself to satisfy someone else's need for control.

One of the first indications of his desire for dominance was how quickly he tried to insert himself into every aspect of my world. Initially, it seemed like he cared deeply about spending time with me. But before long, it became clear that his constant need for attention was not out of love—it was to cut me off from the people who mattered most. If I wanted to talk to friends or family, he would find ways to make me feel guilty, saying things like, "Why do you need them when you have me?" Slowly, I withdrew from my social circle, not realizing that I was being isolated.

He also preyed on my insecurities. Like anyone, I had moments of self-doubt. Instead of supporting me through them, he used those vulnerabilities to tighten his control. "You're lucky I'm here to help you," he would say. "Without me, you'd be lost." At first, I dismissed these remarks, but over time, I started to believe them. I started to think I wasn't capable of success or happiness on my own.

The most telling sign of all was how he reacted whenever I tried to assert myself. Anytime I made a decision without his input, like leasing a vehicle or making plans independently, he would accuse me of being selfish or not prioritizing our relationship. Because I feared losing him, I would back down. Every time I apologized, every time I gave in, I was handing him more control over my life.

I wish I had recognized these behaviors sooner. I wish someone had told me that love and compromise should never make you feel small or scared. By the time I realized how deep his control went, I was already in a situation where I felt trapped.

The Impact of Societal Norms on Recognizing Red Flags

One of the reasons I missed so many of the red flags is because of the way society talks about relationships. We're often told that love is supposed to be intense, that a "good" relationship requires sacrifice. While there's some truth to that, there's a fine line between healthy compromise and toxic control.

In movies and TV shows, relationships are often portrayed as all-consuming, where one person becomes the other's entire world. While that might look romantic on screen, in real life, it's a dangerous dynamic. When one person holds all the power in a relationship, it's not love—it's control.

But these cultural narratives made it hard for me to see what was really happening. I thought that if I loved him, I was supposed to give him all of my time, all of my attention. I believed that putting him first was just part of being in a relationship. At first, it didn't occur to me that I was losing myself in the process.

And it's not just the media that influences how we think about relationships—families and communities play a role too. I grew up hearing phrases like, "Relationships take work," or "You have to make sacrifices for love." So when things started to feel even slightly off in my relationship, I told myself it was normal. I thought that everyone goes through hard times and that maybe I just needed to try harder, be more understanding, or give more of myself.

But the truth is, no one should have to sacrifice their independence or self-worth for love. Love should build you up, not tear you down. And it's only in hindsight that I can see how much I sacrificed for a relationship that was never healthy to begin with.

How Friends and Family Can Miss the Signs

It wasn't just me who missed the red flags—my friends and family missed them too. And that's not to blame them; it's just the reality of emotional and psychological abuse. Often, it's because of the isolation that the signs or red flags are missed. It's easy to overlook them when they're so subtle, so insidious, that even the people closest to you don't see it happening.

In my case, my family thought I was just busy with a new relationship. They didn't realize that I was calling as much because I was being manipulated. When they did start to notice that something was off, I wasn't ready to admit it. I made excuses. I told them I was fine. I convinced myself that they didn't understand how much he cared about me.

My friends saw it too. They noticed that I wasn't friends with them on social media anymore, or that I had blocked them. The friends I was allowed to communicate with didn't see me outside of work, and that I seemed more anxious and less confident. But when they tried to talk to me about it, I brushed them off. I didn't want to hear what they had to say because deep down, I knew they were right, and I wasn't ready to face the truth.

That's the thing about emotional abuse—it makes you feel isolated, not just from the people around you, but from yourself. You start to lose touch with your own reality, and the abuser becomes the only person you feel you can rely on. And because of that, it's incredibly difficult to reach out for help, even when the people who love you are trying to support you.

Breaking Through the Fog of Abuse

The hardest part about recognizing emotional and psychological abuse is that it clouds your judgment. It makes you question everything—your own feelings, your own memories, your own instincts. Because of that, it's easy to stay in the fog of abuse for a long time without realizing how much damage is being done.

For me, breaking through that fog took time. It took small moments of clarity, where I started to see the patterns and recognize the control. It wasn't an overnight realization—it was a slow, very painful process. But eventually, I began to see that what I was experiencing wasn't love. It was manipulation. It was control. It was abuse.

And once I saw it for what it was, I couldn't unsee it. The red flags that I had ignored for so long became impossible to overlook. I started to realize how much of myself I had lost, how much of my life had been shaped by someone else's control.

Recognizing the Unseen Signs

Recognizing the signs of emotional and psychological abuse isn't easy. It's subtle, it's gradual, and it often disguises itself as love or concern. But the signs are there if you know what to look for.

If you're in a relationship that makes you feel small, that makes you doubt yourself, that makes you feel like you're walking on eggshells, those are red flags. If you find yourself apologizing for things that aren't your fault, or if you feel like you need to get your partner's approval for every decision you make, those are signs of control.

And if you're watching a loved one go through something similar, pay attention. Maybe even document what you are seeing or hearing from them. Emotional abuse thrives in silence and secrecy, but with the right support, it can be uncovered. Sometimes, all it takes is someone noticing that something is wrong to start the process of breaking free.

CHAPTER 3

SPOTTING RED FLAGS
IN RELATIONSHIPS

One of the hardest parts of being in an emotionally and psychologically abusive relationship is that the signs often aren't obvious. The abuse often starts small—so small, in fact, that you don't even recognize it for what it is. Yet, when you look back, the red flags were always there, hidden in the normal ups and downs of a relationship.

Understanding Red Flags

Red flags are subtle signals, small indicators that something isn't right. However, because we're often taught to brush off minor issues in relationships as "normal," it's easy to overlook these early signs. And that's exactly what abusers rely on. They count on you dismissing the warning signs, thinking, "It's not a big deal," or, "All couples go through this."

But those red flags? They're not small at all, sometimes they are bright neon flags. They're the early signs of control, manipulation, and abuse. Once you start seeing them for what they are, it's hard to unsee them.

Subtle Signs to Look for: Manipulation, Isolation, Love Bombing, and Controlling Behavior

In my own experience, the red flags started showing up almost immediately. But I ignored the initial red flags because I thought he was a good person, I gave him the benefit of the doubt. They weren't dramatic flags waving to get my attention–there were no big blow-ups, no obvious moments of cruelty. Instead, the red flags were hidden in small actions, subtle comments, and seemingly harmless behaviors.

1. **Manipulation disguised as caring**: One of the first red flags in my relationship was how my partner would manipulate or "groom" me, all while making it seem like he "cared" for me. He'd say things like, "You don't look happy to be here with me" even when I was smiling, and "Your friends and social media disrupt our relationship," or, "I'm only telling you this because I want what's best for you." At first glance, it appeared he was looking out for me. In reality, he was undermining my relationships and making me doubt my own judgment.

2. **Isolation under the guise of love**: Another major red flag was the way he slowly isolated me from the people in my life. He wanted all of my time and attention. Initially, I thought it was because he loved me so much. But over time, I realized that his constant need for attention was a way to cut me off from the support system I needed. I stopped seeing my friends. I stopped having a social life. And before I knew it, he was the only person I had left.

3. **Love bombing**: This tactic is tricky because love bombing feels amazing at first. The abuser showers you with affection, attention, and gifts. You feel like the center of their world. But love bombing isn't about love—it's about control. It's about getting you emotionally hooked so that when the abuse starts, you're already too invested to walk away.

4. **Controlling behavior framed as "advice"**: Another subtle red flag was how he started giving me "advice" about everything in my life—what I wore, how I spent my money, who I communicated with. At first, it didn't seem like control; he framed it as helpful guidance. But over time, his "advice" became more and more controlling, until I felt like I couldn't make a single decision without his approval.

These behaviors can be easy to dismiss, especially in the early stages of a relationship. But they're all signs of control, and they're all designed to make you dependent on the abuser.

Recognizing these red flags early can help prevent you from getting deeper into an abusive relationship.

Behavioral Shifts: When Your Loved One Changes and Becomes More Isolated

One of the most heartbreaking aspects of emotional abuse is how it changes you. I didn't realize it at the time, but I was slowly becoming a different person—a quieter, more fearful version of myself. I used to be outgoing, confident, and independent. But by the time the abuse had taken hold, I was none of those things anymore.

It wasn't just that I was more anxious or less sure of myself; I had also become isolated from the people who could have helped me. I wasn't allowed to reach out to specific friends and I stopped seeing my family as much. When I would see my family all he would do was complain and figure out ways to separate us away from them. My abuser had convinced me that they weren't on our side, that they didn't understand me the way he did.

This isolation is one of the biggest red flags in an abusive relationship. Abusers know that if they can cut you off from your support system, you'll be easier to control. Without friends or family to turn to, you'll be more dependent on them, more likely to stay even when the abuse escalates. This is part of the trauma bond.

If you notice someone you love becoming more isolated—pulling away from friends, canceling plans, or avoiding family—it's worth asking why. They might not be ready to admit what's going on, but just letting them know that you're there for them can make a significant difference.

Common Patterns in Abusers: Controlling Social Media, Financial Control, Jealousy, and Surveillance

Abusers often follow common patterns when it comes to controlling their victims. These patterns can be difficult to spot at first because they're often disguised as concern or love. Over time, these behaviors become more and more obvious, and the control becomes suffocating.

1. **Controlling social media:** One of the first things my abuser did was start monitoring my social media accounts. He wanted to know who I was talking to, what I was posting, and who was commenting on my posts. Initially, I thought it was just protective behavior, but over time, it became clear that this was a way for him to keep tabs on me. He would get angry if I posted something he didn't like, if someone showed up as "someone you may know", or if I talked to someone he didn't approve of.

2. **Financial control:** Another common tactic is controlling the victim's finances. In my case, he started by giving me "advice" on how to spend my money,

insisting and guilting me that it should be for 'us' only. Eventually, he manipulated me out of half of my retirement account for "our" condo. I wasn't allowed to make any financial decisions without his approval, which made it incredibly difficult to leave the relationship.

3. **Jealousy disguised as love**: My abuser was extremely jealous, but he always framed it as love. "I just love you so much, I don't want to share you with anyone else," he would say. At first, it felt flattering, like he cared so much about me that he didn't want anyone else to have my attention. But jealousy isn't love—it's about control. As his jealousy escalated, so did his attempts to isolate me from anyone he saw as a threat.

4. **Surveillance**: Abusers often use surveillance as a way to keep their victims in line. In my case, it started with him checking my phone, but it eventually escalated to him tracking my location and monitoring my online activity–demanding access to my emails, social media, and web search history. He even sent me to work several times without my phone so he had time to dig through its contents. I felt like I couldn't go anywhere or do anything without him knowing about it.

These patterns of control are incredibly common in abusive relationships, and they're all designed to keep the victim dependent on the abuser. If you recognize these behaviors in your own relationship or in the relationship of someone you care about, it's crucial to take action.

Questions to Ask When Something Feels "Off" in Your Loved One's Relationship

If you suspect that someone you love is in an emotionally or psychologically abusive relationship, it's important to approach the situation with care. They might not be ready to discuss what's happening, or they might not even realize they're being abused. However, there are gentle ways to open up the conversation and help them start recognizing the red flags.

Here are some questions to consider asking if you notice that something feels "off" in their relationship:

1. **"How do you feel when you're with them?"**: This question can help your loved one reflect on their feelings. If they hesitate or struggle to answer, it might be a sign that something isn't right.

2. **"Do you feel like you have to change who you are to make them happy?"**: Emotional and psychological abuse often involves making the victim feel inadequate. If your loved one feels like they have to change their personality, appearance, or behavior to keep their partner happy, that's a red flag.

3. **"Do you feel like you can spend time with your friends and family without guilt?"**: Abusers often

try to isolate their victims from their support system. If your loved one feels guilty or anxious about spending time with others, it's worth exploring why.

4. **"Do they make you feel small or insecure?"**: Emotional abusers often use criticism and manipulation to undermine their victims' self-worth. If your loved one is constantly second-guessing themselves or feeling like they're not good enough, itcould be a sign of abuse.

These questions aren't meant to accuse or confront—they're intended to open up a dialogue and help your loved one start recognizing the signs of abuse for themselves. Be patient and understanding, they might not be ready to acknowledge what's happening right away. You can help by documenting their responses, which can be useful when they're away from the abuser.

Conclusion: Seeing the Red Flags for What They Are

Red flags in relationships are easy to miss, especially when they're disguised as love or concern. But once you start to recognize them, they're impossible to ignore. Emotional and psychological abuse thrives in secrecy and silence, but by paying attention to these early warning signs, you can help yourself or a loved one avoid getting trapped in a toxic, controlling relationship.

If you notice any of these behaviors in your own relationship or in the relationship of someone you care about, don't dismiss them. Don't brush them off as "normal" relationship problems. Trust your instincts. If something feels off, it probably is.

Remember, you are not alone. Whether you're experiencing the abuse yourself or trying to help someone else, there are resources and people who can support you. The most crucial step is recognizing the red flags and taking action before things escalate further.

CHAPTER 4

APPROACHING A LOVED ONE IN A CONTROLLING RELATIONSHIP

Talking to someone about their abusive relationship is never easy. It's a conversation filled with emotional landmines, fear, and uncertainty—not just for the victim, but for you as a concerned friend or family member. You don't want to push them away, yet remaining silent while they suffer feels equally unacceptable. Finding the balance is delicate.

When I was in the thick of my emotionally abusive relationship, I remember the well-meaning people who tried to help me. My friends and family could see the red flags before I could. However, every time they approached me, I felt defensive, ashamed, and even more confused. Their words, though filled with love, sometimes pushed me further into the relationship. Why?

Because approaching someone who is being controlled isn't just about what you say—it's about how you say it, when you say it, and most importantly, how much empathy you bring to the conversation.

Let me be clear: it's a challenging conversation to have. When someone is in an emotionally or psychologically abusive relationship, they often don't perceive it the way you do. The abuser has likely twisted their perception of reality, making them feel like the abuse is normal, or worse, making them believe that they are the problem. So, when you approach them, you're not merely trying to help them see the abuse—you're battling the abuser's narrative, which may include gaslighting and manipulation.

For me, it took multiple attempts before I started to see the truth. Each time they reached out, it planted a seed of doubt in my mind. While I wasn't ready to leave in those moments, those seeds eventually grew into the realization that I needed to get out. This chapter is about how to plant those seeds—how to approach a loved one with care, patience, and understanding, while giving them the space to come to their own conclusions.

Understanding the Fear and Confusion Your Loved One May Feel

Before you approach someone in an abusive relationship, it's crucial to understand their internal struggles. From the outside, it might seem obvious to you that they're being controlled, manipulated, or mistreated. But from their perspective, things are murky. Abusers are experts at making their victims feel confused, disoriented, and dependent. In many cases, the victim doesn't recognize the relationship as abusive—or if they do, they feel powerless to change it.

When I was in my relationship, I frequently wavered between wanting to leave and doubting my perceptions. There were moments when I thought, "This isn't right. This isn't how love is supposed to feel." Yet my abuser would always find a way to pull me back in—excusing away his behavior, love-bombing me, or convincing me that I was the one who needed to change. It created a relentless cycle of doubt, guilt, and fear.

One of the biggest reasons victims stay in abusive relationships is due to emotional attachment. This is known as **Trauma Bonding**. Even though they might recognize the harm in the relationship, they still feel love for the person who is hurting them. That emotional connection makes leaving incredibly challenging. The abuser might be controlling, manipulative, and cruel, but they are also the person the victim has shared intimate moments with, relied on for emotional support (however toxic), and, in many cases, the person they believe they can't live without.

In addition to emotional attachment, there's also the fear of the unknown. Leaving an abusive relationship is terrifying; it means stepping into uncertainty. The abuser has often convinced the victim that they won't survive on their own—that they aren't strong enough, smart enough, or capable enough to make it without them. After being beaten down emotionally and psychologically for so long, many start to believe it.

When you approach your loved one, remember that they are likely experiencing a whirlwind of emotions—love, fear, guilt, shame, and confusion, all at once. They might not be ready to face the truth of their situation, and even if they are, they might not feel strong enough to leave. Their abuser may also intervene, further clouding their judgment. Understanding this emotional complexity is key to approaching them in a supportive, non-judgmental manner.

Creating a Safe and Supportive Environment for Conversation

When you're ready to approach your loved one, the first step is to create a safe space for discussion. This conversation cannot be rushed or held in passing; it needs to be intentional, thoughtful, and, most importantly, free from distractions and interruptions.

I remember when a coworker first tried to talk to me about my relationship. We were at lunch, and she casually mentioned that she had noticed changes in me. I immediately became defensive, partly because we were in a public place, and partly because I wasn't ready to admit that something was wrong. It wasn't the right time or setting for such a heavy conversation.

Here are a few key tips for creating a safe and supportive environment:

1. **Choose a private, comfortable setting**: Ensure you're in a place where your loved one feels safe to open up. This could be at home, during a walk in the park, or somewhere they feel relaxed. Avoid public places where they might feel embarrassed or exposed, this can be an emotional discussion.

2. **Be patient and non-confrontational**: The goal is to open up a dialogue, not to accuse or blame. Use a calm and gentle tone and make it clear that you're coming from a place of love and concern.

3. **Start with empathy, not accusations**: Instead of saying, "You're being abused!" or "Your partner is controlling you!" start by expressing how much you care. You might say, "I've noticed you seem a little different lately, and I just want to check in. How are you feeling?" This opens the door for them to share without feeling attacked.

4. **Offer a listening ear, not solutions**: One of the most important things you can do is listen. They might not be ready to hear advice or take action, and that's okay. What they need most in that moment is to feel heard and understood. They want to feel like what they are feeling is valid.

5. **Assure them of confidentiality**: Let them know that whatever they share with you will remain between

you two. They need to trust that they can be honest without fearing judgment or gossip.

By fostering a supportive and non-judgmental environment, you give your loved one the space to open up at their own pace. This conversation isn't about pushing them to leave or take immediate action; it's about helping them begin to see their situation clearly while feeling safe and supported.

Dos and Don'ts: What to Say and What to Avoid

Now that you've created a safe space, the next step is navigating the conversation itself. This is where things can get tricky because, despite your good intentions, certain phrases can unintentionally push your loved one away or make them feel even more trapped. The language you use is crucial.

Here are important **Dos** and **Don'ts** to keep in mind:

Do:

- **Use "I" statements**: Focus on your feelings and observations rather than accusing them or their partner. For instance, say, "I'm worried about you," or "How can I help you or be there for you" instead of, "Your partner is abusive."
- **Express your love and concern**: Let them know that you're coming from a place of care, not judgment. For

example, "I care about you deeply, and I've noticed that you don't seem like yourself lately."

- **Validate their feelings**: If they open up, acknowledge their feelings. Say things like, "That sounds really hard," or "It's understandable that you're feeling confused." Don't minimize their emotions, even if you don't fully understand them.

- **Acknowledge the complexity of the situation**: Recognize that leaving isn't straightforward. Say things like, "I know this is complicated, and I'm here for you no matter what."

Don't:

- **Don't use accusatory language**: Phrases like, "You need to leave," or "Why are you staying with them?" can make your loved one feel defensive. Instead, focus on expressing concern without telling them what to do.

- **Don't criticize the abuser directly**: As tempting as it may be, avoid saying things like, "They're a terrible person," or "How can you be with someone like that?" This can prompt your loved one to defend their partner, shutting down the conversation. If they stay, they may share your comments, isolating you further from their situation. It becomes "You're either for me or against me" in their relationship dynamic and this can become dangerous.

- **Don't pressure them to leave**: Leaving an abusive relationship is a process, and it doesn't happen overnight. Telling them they need immediately can overwhelm them and make them feel stuck.
- **Don't make it about you**: Avoid saying things like, "I can't believe you're letting this happen," or, "I don't understand why you won't listen to me." This conversation isn't about your feelings—it's about helping them feel supported.

Using the right language can significantly influence how the conversation unfolds. Remember, the goal isn't to force them to make a decision immediately—it's to plant a seed of doubt about the relationship and show them know that they have someone in their corner when they're ready.

Real-Life Scenarios and How to Respond Effectively

Let's explore some common scenarios you might encounter when approaching a loved one about their abusive relationship, and how to respond effectively:

Scenario 1: When They Deny the Abuse

Your loved one might not recognize the abuse, or they might not be ready to admit it. If they deny the abuse, don't push them to agree with you. Instead, gently offer examples of what you've noticed and express your concern.

- **What to say**: "I understand that you don't see it that way right now, but I've noticed things that worry me. Like when they criticize you in front of others or get upset when you spend time with friends or have cameras watching your every move. I'm here for you no matter what, and it's ok to talk to me if you ever feel like something's not right."

Scenario 2: When They Acknowledge the Abuse but Are Afraid to Leave

Sometimes, your loved one might admit that they're in an unhealthy or abusive relationship, but they feel trapped or scared to leave. This fear might stem from emotional dependence, financial control, or fear of retaliation. It's important to validate their fear while offering support, without making them feel pressured.

- **What to say**: "I can't imagine how hard this is for you. It must be incredibly confusing to feel like this. I want you to know that I'm here for you, no matter what. You don't have to make any decisions today, but when you're ready to talk about what you want to do, I'll be here to support you every step of the way."
- **What not to say**: "Why don't you just leave? You need to get out of this situation right now." While your

desire to help is genuine, this approach can overwhelm them and make them feel like they're not in control of their own decisions.

In this situation, it's crucial to understand that their fear is real, and leaving an abusive relationship is often more complicated than it seems. Offering reassurance that they don't have to go through it alone can make them feel more empowered to take action when they're ready.

Scenario 3: When They Are Ready to Leave but Don't Know How

If your loved one is ready to leave the relationship but feels unsure of how to do it safely, this is where you can step in with practical support. Leaving an abuser can be dangerous, so it's crucial to help them plan carefully.

- **What to say**: "It's incredible that you've made this decision, and I want to help you do it safely. Let's figure out the next steps together. Have you thought about where you could go or what you'll need? We can create a plan to get you out of there when you feel ready."
- **Offer resources**: Depending on the situation, you can offer to help with things like finding a safe place to stay, gathering important documents, or contacting domestic violence hotlines for professional support.

- **What not to say**: "Just pack your bags and leave tonight." While it might feel like the most straightforward solution, leaving in a rush can escalate the danger, especially if the abuser suspects something is wrong. It's vital to help them leave in a way that minimizes risk and keeps them safe.

Helping them create a safety plan is one of the most practical and impactful things you can do. Make sure they know they can take their time and leave when it's safe to do so, and offer to be there every step of the way.

Scenario 4: When They Have Already Left but Are Emotionally Struggling

Leaving an abusive relationship doesn't mean the struggle is over. The emotional aftermath can be just as challenging, and your loved one may feel lost, overwhelmed, or tempted to return. Your continued support is crucial in this phase.

- **What to say**: "I know this is really hard, and it's okay to feel whatever you're feeling right now. You did something incredibly brave by leaving, but that doesn't mean it will feel easy. I'm here to help you through this, whether it's talking, finding resources, or just being with you when you need company."
- **What not to say**: "At least you're out of the relationship, so you should feel better now." Leaving an abuser

is only the first step in a long healing process, and your loved one may need time, therapy, and ongoing support to rebuild their life.

Even after they leave, the abuser may try to reel them back in through apologies, promises to change, or guilt. The trauma bond created during the relationship can be very powerful. Being there for them emotionally can make all the difference in helping them stay strong and move forward.

Supporting Them While Respecting Their Boundaries

One of the most difficult aspects of supporting someone in an abusive relationship is balancing your desire to help with respecting their autonomy and boundaries. It's natural to want to take control or make decisions for them, but this can often backfire.

Here's how you can support them while respecting their boundaries:

1. **Offer help without taking over**: Let your loved one know that you're there to help, but allow them to make their own decisions. You might say, "I'm here if you ever need to talk, or if you want help finding resources. But I also understand if you're not ready yet."
2. **Respect their pace**: They may not be ready to leave immediately, or they might choose to stay longer than

you'd like. While this can be frustrating, it's vital to respect their timeline and continue offering support without pressure. The more you push, the more they might retreat, especially if they aren't ready to take action.

3. **Consistent support**: One of the most valuable things you can offer is consistency. Let them know that your support isn't conditional on them making a certain decision. Whether they stay or leave, you'll be there for them. This reassures them they have someone to rely on, no matter what.

4. **Avoid judgment**: If they decide to stay in the relationship, try not to show frustration or disappointment. Continue to express empathy and concern. Remember, emotional abuse is complex, and leaving is a process, not a single decision.

5. **Take care of yourself**: Supporting someone in an abusive relationship can take an emotional toll on you, too. Recognize your limits and seek support for yourself if needed. You can't pour from an empty cup, so prioritize your own mental health while helping them.

Ultimately, the goal is to be a lifeline for your loved one without becoming their decision-maker. They need to know that they're in control of their own choices, while your role is support, listen, and help them find their way back to safety.

A Long Journey, But Not Alone

Approaching a loved one who is in a controlling or abusive relationship is one of the most delicate and challenging things you can do. It requires patience, empathy, and a deep understanding of the emotional complexities they're experiencing. It's not just about recognizing the abuse—it's about helping them see it for themselves, in their own time, while offering the support they need to take action when they're ready.

Remember that this is a journey, not a one-time conversation. The seeds you plant today might not take root immediately, but they will eventually grow. Every time you offer a listening ear or demonstrate your care, you help them move one step closer to recognizing the truth of their situation.

And most importantly, remind them that they are not alone. The journey out of an abusive relationship is long and challenging, but with your support and the right resources, they can reach the other side. Sometimes, all it takes is knowing that someone has their back to give them the courage to take that first step.

CHAPTER 5

THE TURNING POINT

E very journey out of an abusive relationship has a critical moment—a turning point when the victim realizes,
"I can't do this anymore. I have to leave." But that realization
doesn't always happen in an instant. For many, it's a series of
small, painful moments that build up over time, eventually leading to the conclusion that staying is no longer an option.

In my own journey, the turning point wasn't marked by a single
dramatic event. Instead, it was a series of moments that chipped
away at my ability to believe the lies my abuser told me—lies
about myself, about our relationship, and about what I deserved.
It was the accumulation of years of manipulation, emotional
abuse, and psychological control that finally pushed me to see
the truth.

Recognizing the turning point is incredibly difficult when you're
in the middle of it. Often, it takes someone outside the relationship—a friend, a family member, a counselor—to help you see
what's really happening. The role of loved ones during this time

is crucial. They can provide the support, clarity, and strength the victim needs to make the decision to leave.

That's what this chapter is about. It's about understanding what the turning point looks like, how to recognize when it's time to act, and how to offer the most effective support during this critical stage of the journey.

Recognizing When It's Time to Act

For many victims, the signs that it's time to leave are evident long before they're ready to admit it. Abusers often escalate their control over time, pushing their victims further and further until something finally snaps. But what does that moment look like? How can you, as a friend or family member, recognize when the victim is nearing that turning point?

Abusers often start small, employing subtle forms of manipulation and control. As the relationship progresses, those tactics escalate. What may have started as harmless requests—like asking the victim to spend more time with them and less with friends—can quickly turn into full-blown isolation, where the victim is cut off from anyone outside the relationship. Control over finances, constant surveillance, and emotional, psychological, and physical abuse follow, causing the victim's sense of self-worth to slowly erode.

Even as the abuse escalates, many victims hold on, convincing themselves that things will improve, that their abuser will change, or that they can fix the relationship if they just try harder. It's only when the control becomes unbearable—when the victim realizes that no amount of effort will change their abuser's behavior—that the turning point arrives.

In my case, it wasn't a single event that made me realize I needed to leave. It was a series of five different times I packed up my belongings and left, only to return and the moments escalated. On last day, the fifth and final time, I found myself sitting on the bed getting told what to do "or else" he would "find someone who would". Why had I stayed so long. The crushing weight of everything I'd been through hit me all at once, and I realized that nothing was ever going to change. That was the turning point for me—the moment I knew I had to get out, even though I was terrified of what leaving would look like.

Key Moments in Tiffiny's Journey

There were several moments in my relationship that, looking back, should have been wake-up calls. But it wasn't until much later that I fully understood what was happening. Like many victims, I made excuses for my abuser, convincing myself that things would get better, that he would change. But the harsh truth is that abusers rarely change; the abuse only escalates.

One of the first key moments for me was realizing how much of myself I had lost. I used to be confident, independent, and full of life. After years of being in a controlling relationship, I hardly recognized myself. I became anxious, constantly second-guessing myself, and walking on eggshells around my partner. I had become a shell of my former self, and I didn't even see it happening.

Another pivotal moment came when I recognized my isolation. My abuser had systematically cut me off from my friends and family–not all at once—but gradually. First, he'd make negative comments about my friends, claiming they didn't care about me or respect our relationship. Then, he discouraged me from spending time with them. Eventually, he demanded I stop seeing them altogether, making excuses or guilting me. It wasn't until I was completely alone that I realized what had happened.

The true turning point for me—the moment that truly made me realize I needed to leave—was when I began to feel like I was losing my mind. My abuser was gaslighting me, making me question my own memories and perceptions. I felt like I couldn't trust myself anymore, and that was terrifying. Sitting in our condo after an argument, that I realized I couldn't live like this anymore. I had to get out.

How Loved Ones Can Help During the Most Critical Stages

When someone reaches their turning point, they need support more than ever. However, it's not always easy to know how to help. This is a delicate time, and while the victim may be ready to leave, they're also dealing with a lot of fear, confusion, and doubt. Here's how you can support them during these critical stages:

1. **Recognize the signs that they're ready to leave**: If your loved one starts expressing unhappiness, mentions feeling trapped, or voices doubts about the relationship, these are signs that they may be nearing their turning point. Pay attention to these signals and be ready to offer support when they're ready to take action.

2. **Offer practical help**: One of the most important things you can do is offer tangible support. This could mean helping them find a safe place to stay, providing financial assistance if they need it, or gathering important documents (like IDs, bank statements, and legal paperwork) before they leave. Even small acts, like offering to watch their kids or helping them pack, can make a huge difference.

3. **Help them create a safety plan**: Leaving an abusive relationship can be dangerous, especially if the abuser is controlling or violent. It's crucial to help your loved one create a safety plan which might involve deciding

where they'll go, how they'll leave without the abuser finding out, and what steps they'll take to stay safe after leaving. Connecting them with local domestic violence hotlines or organizations that specialize in safety planning can be invaluable.

4. **Stay patient and supportive, even if they hesitate**: Victims often waver, even after deciding to leave. Their abuser has typically created an alternate reality for them, leading to self-doubt and hesitation. If your loved one seems uncertain, refrain from showing frustration or pressure. Instead, reassure them of your support, no matter how long it takes.

5. **Offer emotional support**: Leaving an abusive relationship is emotionally exhausting. Your loved one may experience a range of feelings—relief, fear, guilt, sadness, and confusion. Let them know that it's okay to feel all of these things and that you're there to listen without judgment.

Lessons Learned: Effective Support and Where Family and Friends Can Improve

In my experience, the support of my loved ones was essential to my decision to leave my abusive relationship. However, there were also moments where well-meaning friends and family unintentionally made things harder. Here are some lessons I've

learned about what works—and what doesn't—when supporting someone in an abusive relationship:

1. **What worked for me**: The people who helped me
   the most were those who didn't pressure me. They
   didn't force me to see the abuse or push me to leave
   before I was ready. Instead, they listened. They offered
   support without judgment, allowing me to come to
   my own conclusions. This made me feel safe and gave
   me the space I needed to make the decision to leave on
   my own terms.

2. **Common mistakes loved ones make**: One of the
   biggest missteps is being too forceful. It's understandable to want to help someone you care about but
   pushing the victim to leave before they're ready can
   backfire, making them feel defensive, ashamed, or even
   more dependent on their abuser. Another common
   mistake is speaking negatively about the abuser. While
   this may seem like a natural reaction, it can make
   the victim feel like they need to defend their partner,
   which can shut down the conversation.

3. **How to avoid these mistakes**: Rather than telling
   the victim what to do, focus on offering support and
   understanding. Ask open-ended questions like, "How
   do you feel when you're with them?" or "What would
   you like to happen next?" or "How can I help?" These
   types questions help the victim reflect on their situation without feeling pressured or judged.

How to Prepare for Difficult Conversations and Stay Strong

Supporting someone in an abusive relationship isn't easy; it takes emotional strength, patience, and resilience. Before you have difficult conversations with your loved one, it's important to prepare yourself emotionally. Here are some tips for staying strong and supportive during these tough moments:

1. **Manage your own emotions**: It's normal to feel angry, frustrated, or sad when you see someone you love being hurt. However, keeping those emotions in check during conversations is crucial. If you come across as overly emotional, they might feel overwhelmed or defensive. Take a deep breath, and remind yourself that this conversation is about them, not you.

2. **Stay calm, even when emotions run high**: Your loved one may react with anger, denial, or sadness when you bring up the abuse or the abuser. It's vital to remain calm, even if the conversation gets heated. If you feel yourself getting upset, take a step back and refocus on your goal: offering support.

3. **Stay firm in your support**: Even if your loved one struggles with doubt or wavers in their decision, maintain your support. Let them know that you believe in them, that you trust their judgment, and willl be there for them no matter what. This kind of unwavering support can give them the strength they need to take the next steps.

The Power of the Turning Point

The turning point is a critical moment in the journey out of an abusive relationship. It's the moment when the victim realizes they deserve better—when they see the abuse for what it is and begin to take steps toward freedom. As a loved one, your role in this moment is crucial. You have the power to offer support, guidance, and reassurance when they need it most.

However, it's important to remember this process is delicate. The turning point isn't always clear-cut, and it's essential to remain patient, understanding, and supportive, even if the victim hesitates or struggles with doubt. By offering consistent, compassionate support, you can help your loved one find the courage to leave and begin the long journey of healing.

Most importantly, remind them that they are not alone. The path out of an abusive relationship is challenging, but with your support—and the support of others—they can make it to the other side. Encourage them to take it one step at a time, celebrating each small victory along the way, and reassure them that healing is a journey.

CHAPTER 6

PROVIDING SAFE SUPPORT WITHOUT JUDGMENT

S upporting someone in an abusive relationship is one of the most delicate and complex challenges. Emotional abuse, particularly coercive control, often runs deeper than people realize. It's not always about physical violence; the abuser manipulates multiple aspects of the victim's life, from their finances to their legal standing, leaving them feeling both dependent and trapped. Recognizing the signs of coercive control is vital, as it includes behaviors like excessive monitoring of communications, isolating the victim from friends and family, and enforcing strict rules about personal choices. While your instinct might be to encourage your loved one to leave the relationship, remember that coercive control can make it difficult for them to see their situation clearly.

In my case, the manipulation extended far beyond emotional abuse to include financial control, surveillance, and legal interference. One instance stands out: my abuser orchestrated a situation that created a need to hire an attorney to remove a photo someone had posted of me on social media. He didn't like how I was dealing with the attorney requests, so he controlled the entire process, using it as another tool to assert his dominance over me, even through legal channels against people I knew.

Understanding the Scope of Abuse

It's essential to understand that the control exerted by abusers can touch unexpected areas of a victim's life. Helping someone leave an abusive relationship isn't as simple as telling them to walk away—it involves untangling a web of manipulation that may include financial dependence, legal complexities, and social isolation.

The Balance of Support

Offering support requires a delicate balance. You want to help them recognize the abuse and encourage them to leave, but you must also be careful not to overwhelm them with advice or push them too hard. There's a fine line between offering help and unintentionally making them feel judged.

After my experience, comments like, "How could you let him treat you that way?" or "You're too strong to stay in a relationship like that" were intended to empower me, but they only deepened my shame and made me feel even more isolated. Instead of feeling supported, I felt as though I had to justify my actions and decisions.

The Challenge of Judgement

That's the challenge of supporting someone in an abusive relationship: if you come across as judgmental, even unintentionally, it can drive them further into the abuser's control. They may feel misunderstood or, worse, start believing the abuse is their fault, making it even harder for them to break free.

How to Offer Emotional and Practical Support

When someone you care about is in an abusive relationship, your first instinct may be to fix the problem. You want to protect them, rescue them, and take them away from the situation. But the truth is, leaving an abusive relationship is a process that must be done on their terms. The best way to help is to offer both emotional and practical support while allowing them to take the lead.

1. **Listening without judgment or pushing for immediate action**: One of the most powerful things you can do is simply listen. Victims of abuse are often

isolated and feel like they have no one to talk to. The abuser often minimizes their feelings, leaving them silenced for so long. By listening—really listening— you give them a chance to express their feelings and fears without judgment.

- ○ **What to say**: "I'm here to listen whenever you're ready to talk. You don't have to make any decisions right now—I just want you to know that you are not alone." or "I can see how hard this is for you, and it's okay to feel confused." Empower them to make their own decisions and gently encourage them to explore their situation more deeply, perhaps suggesting they speak with a professional who understands the dynamics of coercive control.
- ○ **What not to say**: "Why haven't you left yet?" or "You need to get out of there." While it's understandable to feel frustrated or worried, pushing them to take action before they're ready can make them feel even more trapped.

2. **Helping with logistical and practical needs**: Emotional support is essential, but practical ways to help can make a huge difference. Many victims of abuse face logistical challenges that make it difficult for them to leave, such as financial dependence, lack of housing, children and/or animals, or fear of legal consequences. Offering practical support can make a huge difference.

○ **Financial support**: If your loved one is financially dependent on their abuser, they may
feel like they can't afford to leave. Offering
temporary financial assistance—covering the
cost of rent, helping them set up a separate
bank account, or providing a loan—can give
them the freedom to make decisions without
fear of financial ruin.

○ **Housing and legal assistance**: Finding a
safe place to stay is often one of the biggest
challenges for victims, especially if they are
escaping with children or pets. Offer to help
them find housing—whether that's staying
with you temporarily, looking for a shelter,
or finding affordable housing options. Legal
assistance may also be necessary for issues
with custody, restraining orders, or divorce.
Connecting them with a lawyer or legal aid
organization can be incredibly helpful.

○ **Safety planning**: Helping your loved one
create a safety plan is another practical way to
offer support. This personalized plan includes
ways to stay safe while in the relationship,
planning to leave, or after leaving. It could
involve identifying a safe place to go, gathering
important documents, and figuring out how
to safely leave without the abuser noticing.

3. **Ensuring their safety while respecting their autonomy**: While offering help, it's crucial to respect their autonomy. It's tempting to take over and make decisions for them, but doing so can unintentionally replicate the control their abuser has over them. Instead, ask how they want to be supported and what they feel comfortable doing.

   ○ **What to say**: "I want to help in whatever way feels right for you. Let me know what you need, and we can figure out the next steps together." Everyone is different and the extent of their needs varies.

   ○ **What not to say**: "Here's what we're going to do. You need to follow this plan." Even if you have good intentions, taking control of the situation can make them feel even more powerless.

Respecting Boundaries: How to Offer Help Without Taking Over

One of the most important things to remember when supporting someone in an abusive relationship is that they need to feel in control of their own decisions. After being in a relationship where their choices and autonomy have been taken away, the last thing they need is for someone else to take over.

It's important to offer help without making them feel like they're losing control of the situation. This means respecting their boundaries, even if they choose to stay in the relationship longer than you'd like.

1. **Why it's important for victims to feel in control of their decisions:** Being in an abusive relationship often means that the victim has lost their sense of agency. They may feel like they have no control over their life, their decisions, or their future. By allowing them to make their own choices—whether that's staying in the relationship for now, or deciding when and how to leave—you're helping them regain a sense of power.

2. **Knowing when to step back:** It can be incredibly difficult to watch someone you love stay in an abusive relationship, but it's important to respect their boundaries and know when to step back. If they're not ready to leave, pushing them to take action can backfire. Instead, let them know that you'll be there for them when they're ready, and continue to offer emotional support.

3. **Practical ways to offer assistance without overstepping:** Instead of making decisions for them, ask how you can help. For example, "Would it help if I found some housing options for you to consider?" or "Would you like me to come with you if you decide

to speak to a lawyer?" Offering options rather than directives allows them to remain in control.

When to Step Back: Avoiding Codependency and Enabling

As much as you want to help, it's important to recognize the line between healthy support and codependency. When you become too involved, you risk enabling the situation or creating an unhealthy dynamic. Here's how to avoid codependency and maintain healthy boundaries:

1. **Understanding codependency and how it can harm both parties**: Codependency happens when one person becomes overly reliant on another for emotional or practical support. In abusive situations, this can manifest when the supporter feels responsible for the victim's well-being. While it's natural to want to help, becoming too enmeshed can lead to burnout and prevent the victim from regaining their independence.

2. **The difference between healthy support and enabling**: Healthy support involves offering help while encouraging the victim to take steps toward independence. Enabling, on the other hand, happens when you take over their responsibilities or make decisions for them. For example, if you find yourself constantly bailing them out of financial or emotional crises without encouraging long-term solutions, you may be enabling the situation.

3. **Signs that you might be over-involved and how to reset boundaries**: If you find yourself feeling overwhelmed, resentful, or emotionally drained by the situation, it might be a sign that you're too involved. To reset boundaries, have an open conversation about what you're able to offer and what you can't. Let them know that you're there to support them, but that you also need to take care of your own well-being.

Taking Care of Yourself While Helping Someone in Crisis

Supporting someone in an abusive relationship can be emotionally exhausting. It's easy to neglect your own needs while caught up in their crisis. But if you don't take care of yourself, you won't be able to offer the support they need. Here are some tips for maintaining your own well-being while helping a loved one:

1. **Set emotional boundaries**: Establish clear emotional boundaries so that you don't become overwhelmed by their situation. This might mean deciding when and how often you'll be available to talk, or recognizing when you need to step back.

2. **Seek your own support**: It's okay to seek help for yourself, too. Whether it's talking to a therapist, joining a support group for loved ones of abuse survivors, or confiding in a trusted friend, having your own support system can help you manage the emotional toll.

3. **Practice self-care**: Taking care of yourself physically, emotionally, and mentally is crucial. Make time for activities that recharge you, whether that's exercise, meditation, spending time with friends, or simply taking a break from the situation.

Recognizing When Professional Help Is Needed

While your support is invaluable, there are times when professional help is necessary. If your loved one is dealing with severe emotional trauma, safety concerns, or legal issues, connecting them with professionals can make all the difference.

1. **Knowing when it's time to involve a counselor, therapist, or legal professional**: If your loved one struggles with mental health issues, such as depression, anxiety, or PTSD, even Complex-PTSD, encouraging them to seek professional help is essential. A counselor or therapist can provide the tools they need to process their trauma and begin healing.

2. **The importance of connecting your loved one with domestic violence organizations**: Domestic violence organizations offer a wide range of services, from emergency housing to legal assistance and counseling. Connecting your loved one with these resources can provide them with the support they need to leave the relationship safely.

3. **How to support someone through therapy or legal processes**: If your loved one decides to seek therapy or pursue legal action, continue to offer emotional support. Encourage them to attend therapy sessions or court hearings and let them know that you're proud of them for taking steps toward healing.

The Power of Non-Judgmental Support

Providing safe support without judgment is one of the most powerful things you can do for someone in an abusive relationship. It requires patience, empathy, and a deep understanding of their emotional and psychological state. By offering both emotional and practical support, respecting their boundaries, and knowing when to step back, you can help them regain their sense of autonomy and strength.

Remember, you can't fix the situation for them, but you can be a steady presence in their life as they navigate their way out of the abuse. Most importantly, take care of yourself throughout this journey. Supporting someone in crisis is hard work, but with the right balance of care and boundaries, you can make a meaningful difference in their life. The goal is to empower them to make choices that lead to their safety and well-being, fostering resilience and independence along the way.

CHAPTER 7

REBUILDING SELF-WORTH AND SETTING BOUNDARIES

Leaving an abusive relationship is an enormous step that requires immense courage, but it's only the beginning of the healing journey. What comes next is often just as challenging–rebuilding your self-worth, regaining your independence, and learning how to live without the constant presence of control and manipulation. For many survivors of emotional and psychological abuse, the damage lingers long after the relationship ends. The scars may not be visible, but they run deep.

I know this firsthand. After leaving my relationship, I didn't just feel free—I felt lost. For so long, I had been defined by someone else's control and manipulation, their constant barrage of criticism and guilt. Without that toxic relationship, I didn't know who I was anymore. My confidence was shattered. My sense of self-worth was nonexistent. I had spent so long being told that

I wasn't good enough, smart enough, or strong enough, and I began to believe it.

Emotional and psychological abuse breaks you down slowly, piece by piece, until you no longer recognize the person you once were. Once you've left, you're faced with the daunting task of putting yourself back together.

But here's the good news—you can rebuild. You can regain your sense of self, your confidence, and your independence. It takes time, patience, and a lot of hard work, but it's possible. I'm living proof of that. In this chapter, we're going to explore how to begin the process of rebuilding your self-worth after emotional and psychological abuse, and why setting boundaries is a critical part of that journey.

The Role of Self-Esteem in Preventing and Overcoming Abuse

Self-esteem is one of the first casualties in an abusive relationship. Abusers typically target their victim's confidence and sense of self-worth because they know that a person with low self-esteem is easier to control. If you don't believe in yourself—if you don't think you're worthy of love, respect, or kindness—it becomes much harder to stand up for yourself or leave a toxic situation.

In my own relationship, my abuser was relentless in his efforts to chip away at my self-esteem. He made comments about my appearance, my intelligence, and my abilities. He would expect me to post on social media proclaiming "I'm so lucky I'm with him." He would say, "No one else would put up with your nonsense." Over time, those comments began to sink in. I started to believe that I was, in fact, lucky to have him. I thought that maybe I wasn't good enough, or I was being too difficult, for anyone else.

That's how emotional abuse works—it makes you doubt yourself and convinces you that you're incapable of living independently or making your own decisions. Once your self-esteem has been eroded, the abuser's control becomes even more powerful.

However, self-esteem can be rebuilt. Just as it was slowly chipped away, it can be gradually restored. Once you begin to rebuild your confidence, you become stronger. You start to realize that you're worthy of love, respect, and kindness—and that you don't need anyone else's approval to feel good about yourself.

Rebuilding self-esteem is crucial in overcoming emotional abuse because it enables you to break free from the cycle of manipulation and control. Without a strong sense of self-worth, it's easy to fall back into old patterns or find yourself in another abusive relationship. But when you have a solid sense of self-worth, you can set boundaries, demand respect, and protect yourself from manipulation.

Recognizing and Healing from the Damage

The first step in rebuilding self-worth is recognizing how emotional and psychological abuse has affected you. This can be difficult because, during the relationship, you may not have fully grasped the extent of the damage. Abusers are skilled at making their victims feel like they're the problem, and you may have internalized much of that blame.

For me, the realization came slowly. After I left, I started to notice how many of my thoughts and behaviors were still shaped by the abuse. I constantly second-guessed myself, even over small decisions. I was afraid to assert myself because I had been conditioned to believe that my opinions didn't matter. I felt guilty for wanting things for myself because I had been taught that my needs were always secondary to his.

It took time to recognize these patterns, but once I did, I could start the healing process. Here are a few steps that helped me begin to rebuild my confidence and self-worth:

1. **Acknowledge the abuse**: The first step is acknowledging that what you went through was abuse. This can be incredibly difficult, especially if the abuse wasn't physical, but validating your experience is essential. Emotional and psychological abuse is just as real and damaging as physical abuse, and acknowledging it is the first step toward healing.

2. **Practice self-compassion**: One of the hardest parts of rebuilding self-worth is learning to be kind to yourself and forgive yourself. After being in an abusive relationship, negative self-talk can be overwhelming. It's important to challenge these thoughts and replace them with self-compassion. Remind yourself that the abuse wasn't your fault, and that you deserve love and respect.

3. **Reclaim your independence**: One of the most empowering things you can do after leaving an abusive relationship is to reclaim your independence. This might mean taking control of your finances, making decisions on your own, or pursuing hobbies and interests that you gave up during the relationship. Rebuilding your independence helps you regain a sense of agency and control over your life.

4. **Seek therapy or support**: Healing from emotional and psychological abuse is a long process, and it's often helpful to seek professional support. A therapist can help you work through the trauma of the abuse and provide you with tools to rebuild your self-esteem. Support groups can also be invaluable, connecting you with others who have had similar experiences.

Healing from emotional abuse isn't linear, and it's important to be patient with yourself. There will be setbacks, but with time and effort, you can rebuild your confidence and start to feel like yourself again.

How to Help Your Loved One Regain Confidence and Independence

If you're supporting someone who has recently left an abusive relationship, one of the most important things you can do is help them rebuild their self-worth. Here are a few ways you can offer support:

1. **Encourage their independence**: One of the most empowering things for someone recovering from abuse is reclaiming their independence. Encourage your loved one to make decisions for themselves, pursue their own interests, and take control of their life. This might start with small decisions, giving them confidence in who they are.

2. **Offer validation and support**: One of the most damaging aspects of emotional abuse is that it makes the victim doubt themselves. Offering validation—reminding them that their feelings are valid and that they're capable of making their own decisions—can help them rebuild their confidence.

3. **Celebrate small victories**: Rebuilding self-worth takes time, and it's important to celebrate the small victories along the way. Whether it's speaking up in a meeting, setting a boundary with someone, or taking a step toward a personal goal, acknowledging and celebrating these moments can help your loved one recognize their progress.

4. **Be patient**: Healing from emotional abuse is a long process, and there will be setbacks. It's important to be patient and understanding, offering support without pushing them to move faster than they're ready.

Tiffiny's Testimony: During my recovery, the people who helped me the most were the ones who believed in me even when I didn't believe in myself. They encouraged me to take small steps toward independence, validated my feelings, and celebrated my progress without judgment. That kind of support was invaluable in helping me rebuild my confidence.

Recognizing Your Own Vulnerabilities: Why Anyone Can Fall Victim to Manipulation

A common misconception is that only "weak" or "naive" people fall victim to emotional abuse. But the truth is, anyone can be manipulated by an abuser, regardless of how strong or independence. Abusers don't target weakness—they target vulnerability, and everyone has vulnerabilities.

In my case, I was independent and confident before my relationship, but I had vulnerabilities that my abuser exploited. I was empathetic, trusting, and eager to please, which he used those against me. He made me feel like I was the only person who truly understood him, and he manipulated my desire to be a good partner into a weapon of control.

It's important to recognize that emotional abuse isn't a reflection of the victim's strength or intelligence—it's a reflection of the abuser's tactics. Abusers are skilled at identifying and exploiting vulnerabilities, using love, affection, loyalty and trust as tools of manipulation.

By recognizing your own vulnerabilities and understanding how abusers operate, you can protect yourself from falling into similar patterns in the future. This doesn't mean closing yourself off or becoming cynical—it means being aware of your boundaries and learning to recognize red flags before they escalate.

Empowering Yourself and Others with Boundaries and Healthy Relationships

One of the most important parts of recovery is learning to set and maintain healthy boundaries. Boundaries are essential for protecting your emotional well-being and preventing future manipulation. For many survivors of abuse, boundaries can feel foreign or difficult to establish—especially if they've been conditioned to believe that their needs don't matter.

Here's how to start setting healthy boundaries:

1. **Identify your needs and limits**: The first step in setting boundaries is identifying your needs and limits. This might involve acknowledging when you need space, when certain behaviors make you

uncomfortable, or when you need to say "no." Take
time to reflect on what you need and be honest with
yourself about what you're willing to tolerate.

2. **Communicate your boundaries clearly**: Once
   you've identified your boundaries, it's essential to
   communicate them clearly to others. This can be
   challenging, especially if you're used to prioritizing
   others' needs over your own. However, asserting your
   boundaries is crucial for maintaining healthy relationships. For example, if someone is being disrespectful,
   you might say, "I don't appreciate being spoken to that
   way, and I'd like for it to stop." Or I won't continue
   this conversation if you continue to speak to me
   like that."

3. **Enforce your boundaries**: Setting boundaries is only
   part of the process—you also need to enforce them.
   This means being consistent and standing firm when
   someone crosses a boundary. If someone disrespects
   your limit, don't hesitate to assert yourself or distance
   yourself from the situation.

4. **Teach others to set boundaries**: One of the most
   powerful ways to break the cycle of abuse is to teach
   others, especially young people, how to set and maintain healthy boundaries. This can involve having open
   conversations about consent, respect, and communication in relationships.

Rebuilding a Stronger, More Confident You

Rebuilding self-worth after emotional and psychological abuse is a long and difficult journey, but it's also one of the most empowering things you can do. By taking small steps to regain your confidence, reclaim your independence, and set healthy boundaries, you can create a life that is free from manipulation and control.

Remember, this process takes time. Be patient with yourself, and don't hesitate to seek support from loved ones, therapists, or support groups. You deserve to feel confident, strong, and in control of your own life. With time and effort, you can rebuild a version of yourself that is stronger and more resilient than ever before.

CHAPTER 8

PREVENTING (OR STOPPING) ABUSE BEFORE IT HAPPENS

One of the hardest lessons I learned from my experience is that prevention is key. I wish I had known what to look for before entering my relationship, but like so many others, I didn't recognize the red flags until it was too late. Emotional and psychological abuse doesn't start out with obvious signs; it begins with subtle manipulation, disguised as love and care. But if I had been educated about those early signs, maybe I could have saved myself years of pain and struggle.

That's why prevention matters. Emotional abuse often escalates gradually, making it easy to dismiss early warning signs as normal relationship behavior. By educating ourselves and others—especially young people—about these red flags, we can stop abuse before it starts. We can empower individuals to recognize manipulation, control, and toxic behavior early on, before they become trapped in an abusive relationship.

In this chapter, we will explore how emotional and psychological abuse can be prevented. We'll look at the early warning signs to watch for, how to educate young people about healthy boundaries, and the steps we can take to build strong, healthy relationships. Prevention is always better than cure, and by learning to spot the signs of abuse before it occurs, we can protect ourselves and our loved ones from years of suffering.

Red Flags to Watch for Before Entering a Relationship

Emotional and psychological abuse doesn't happen overnight. It starts small, with subtle signs that, if left unchecked, can escalate into something much more dangerous. The challenge is that these early signs are often easy to dismiss, especially when a new relationship feels exciting.

In my own relationship, the red flags were there from the very beginning, yet I failed to see them for what they were. My abuser was charming, attentive, and made me feel like the most important person in the world. However, over time, his charm morphed into control, his attention became suffocating, and his love felt more like possession.

Here are some of the early red flags I wish I had known to look for:

1. **Love bombing**: One of the first signs of an emotionally and psychologically abusive relationship is love
   bombing. This is when the abuser overwhelms you
   with affection, attention, gifts, and compliments early
   on. Initially, it feels amazing—like you've found someone who truly "gets you", and values you. However,
   love bombing is often a tactic to create emotional
   dependence before the abuse begins. Once they have
   you, the behavior changes, and the love bombing is
   replaced by control and manipulation.

2. **Excessive jealousy and possessiveness**: Jealousy can
   be mistaken for care, but excessive jealousy is a major
   red flag. If your partner becomes upset when you talk
   to others, accuses you of flirting, or tries to control
   who you spend time with, that's not love—that's
   control. In my relationship, the jealousy started out
   with small comments and escalated to the point where
   I wasn't "allowed" to talk to certain people or go places
   without his approval.

3. **Isolation from friends and family**: Abusers often
   try to isolate their victims from their support systems.
   This might begin with your partner questioning why
   you need to spend so much time with friends or family,
   or making you feel guilty for wanting to be around
   others. Over time, they might try to cut you off from
   your loved ones entirely, making you more dependent on them. If your partner is discouraging you or

guilting you from seeing friends or family, that's a significant red flag.

4. **Constant need for reassurance**: Emotional abusers often require constant validation from their partners. They might ask you to prove your love repeatedly, or make you feel like you're not doing enough to show how much you care. In my relationship, my partner would constantly ask, "Are you happy to be here with me?" even when I was smiling or, "Why didn't you text me the second you got home or got to work?" It felt like nothing I did was ever enough.

5. **Subtle put-downs disguised as jokes**: A common tactic abusers use is to make hurtful comments and then dismiss them as "just jokes." They might tease you about your appearance, intelligence, or abilities in a way that feels uncomfortable. When you call them out on it, they'll say you're overreacting. This is a form of emotional manipulation, designed to chip away at your self-esteem.

Recognizing these red flags early can save you from getting deeper into a toxic relationship. If you notice any of these behaviors in a new partner, it's important to address them right away, or even consider walking away before things escalate.

Educating Young People About Manipulation and Setting Healthy Boundaries

One of the most important preventative measures against emotional abuse is educating young people about healthy relationships. Too often, teenagers and young adults enter into their first relationships without understanding the distinction between love and control, or between healthy attention and manipulation. By starting these conversations early, we can help young people recognize the signs of toxic behavior and empower them to set boundaries.

When I was growing up, no one discussed emotional abuse with me. I didn't know what manipulation looked like, and I didn't understand that love could be used as a weapon of control. I entered my relationship completely unprepared for the red flags that now seem so obvious. That's why it's vital to engage young people in these discussions before they find themselves in unhealthy relationships.

Here are a few key lessons that can help young people recognize manipulation and set healthy boundaries:

1. **Teach about consent and respect**: Consent isn't just about physical boundaries—it's about emotional boundaries too. Young people need to understand that in a healthy relationship, both partners respect each other's boundaries and make decisions together.

If one partner is constantly pushing the other's limits or trying to control their actions, that's a sign of an unhealthy relationship.

2. **Discuss love bombing and manipulation**: Many teenagers misinterpret love bombing for genuine affection. They believe that someone who showers them with attention and affection truly loves them. It's essential to teach them that love bombing is often a tactic used by abusers to create emotional dependence. Recognizing this behavior early can help young people avoid falling into the trap of emotional manipulation.

3. **Encourage setting and enforcing boundaries**: One of the most powerful tools we can give young people is the ability to set and enforce boundaries. This means teaching them that it's okay to say "no," to take time for themselves, and to demand respect in their relationships. It's also important to teach them that if someone disrespects their boundaries, it's a red flag and a reason to reconsider the relationship.

4. **Model healthy relationships**: Young people often learn about relationships by observing the adults around them. By modeling healthy relationships—whether that's with a partner, friends, or family members—you can demonstrate what respect, communication, and mutual support look like. Witnessing healthy relationships in action equips them to recognize toxic behavior when it occurs.

By initiating these conversations early, we can empower young people to make informed decisions about their relationships and protect themselves from emotional and psychological abuse.

Recognizing and Addressing Toxic Behavior in Friendships and Family Relationships

Emotional abuse doesn't only occur in romantic relationships; it can also manifest in friendships and family dynamics. Many of the same red flags we see in abusive romantic relationships also appear in toxic friendships and family relationships, but they're often harder to spot because we don't think of those relationships in the same way.

In my own life, I've seen toxic behavior in friendships and work relationships that mirrored the control and manipulation I experienced in my romantic relationship. Friends or coworkers who consistently criticized me, made me feel guilty for asserting my boundaries, or tried to control my decisions were engaging in emotionally abusive behaviors.

Here are some signs of toxic behavior to watch for in friendships, work, and family relationships:

1. **Constant criticism and judgment**: A toxic friend, co-worker, or family member may frequently put you down or criticize your choices. They might make you feel inadequate or as though you're always in the

wrong. This is a form of emotional manipulation, designed to make you doubt yourself and feel dependent on their approval.

2. **Guilt-tripping**: Toxic individuals often use guilt to control you. They may make you feel guilty for not spending enough time with them, for asserting your boundaries, or for not living up to their expectations. This can hinder your ability to prioritize your own needs or make decisions that are best for you.

3. **Control over your decisions**: Just like in romantic relationships, toxic friends, co-workers, and family members may try to control your decisions. They might pressure you into doing things you're not comfortable with, or make you feel obligated to prioritize their needs over your own. This creates an unhealthy dynamic where you feel trapped or obligated to please them.

4. **Emotional manipulation**: Toxic individuals might use emotional manipulation to achieve their goals. This could involve playing the victim, using passive-aggressive behavior, or making you feel responsible for their happiness. Over time, this can erode your self-esteem and make you feel like you're walking on eggshells around them.

If you recognize any of these behaviors in your friendships, work or family relationships, it's essential to address them. Setting boundaries with toxic individuals can be challenging, but it's crucial for protecting your emotional well-being. If the person refuses to respect your boundaries, it may be necessary to distance yourself from the relationship.

How to Help Loved Ones Regain Their Sense of Worth After Abuse

After experiencing emotional abuse, rebuilding one's sense of worth is crucial. This can be a lengthy and challenging process, but with the right support, it's possible to regain confidence and independence.

If you're helping a loved one recover from emotional abuse, here are some steps you can take to support them:

1. **Encourage self-reflection and self-awareness**: One of the first steps in rebuilding self-worth is recognizing how the abuse affected them. Encourage your loved one to reflect on their experiences and how the relationship made them feel. This can be done through journaling–writing about what they remember, how they felt during specific situations, and how they feel now since they have escaped. This process can help them gain a deeper understanding of what happened and reinforce that it wasn't their fault.

2. **Validate their feelings**: Emotional abuse often leaves victims feeling as though their emotions don't matter. As a supportive friend or family member, one of the

most vital things you can do is validate their feelings. Let them know that their emotions are legitimate and that it's okay to feel angry, sad, or confused. This validation can help them start to rebuild their self-esteem.

3. **Celebrate small victories**: Recovery from emotional abuse doesn't happen overnight. It's important to celebrate small victories along the way. Whether it's setting a boundary, taking a step toward independence, or simply recognizing their own worth, acknowledging these milestones can help your loved one see their progress.

4. **Encourage them to seek professional support**: While your support is invaluable, it's equally important to encourage your loved one to seek professional help if they need it. A therapist can provide the tools they need to process their trauma and rebuild their confidence.

The Importance of Self-Awareness in Building Strong, Healthy Relationships

One of the most powerful tools for preventing future abuse is self-awareness. When you understand your own triggers, vulnerabilities, and patterns, you're better equipped to protect yourself from manipulation and control.

Here's how self-awareness can help you build strong, healthy relationships:

1. **Recognizing your own patterns**: Many of us have relationship patterns we aren't even aware of. Perhaps you tend to prioritize your partner's needs over your own, or you often ignore red flags because you don't want to be alone. By recognizing these patterns, you can make conscious decisions to change them.

2. **Understanding your vulnerabilities**: We all have vulnerabilities, whether it's a fear of abandonment, a desire for approval, or a need for control. Abusers often exploit these vulnerabilities, so it's crucial to understand what they are. By becoming aware of your own vulnerabilities, you can take steps to protect yourself from manipulation.

3. **Developing emotional intelligence**: Emotional intelligence is the ability to recognize, understand, and manage your own emotions, as well as those of others. Developing emotional intelligence can help you navigate relationships more effectively and protect yourself from toxic behavior.

By building self-awareness, you can create stronger, healthier relationships that are based on mutual respect, trust, and communication.

Taking Steps Toward Prevention

Preventing emotional and psychological abuse before it occurs is possible, but it requires education, self-awareness, and a commitment to setting healthy boundaries. By recognizing red flags early, educating young people about manipulation, and fostering strong relationships grounded in respect, we can protect ourselves and our loved ones from the pain of abuse.

Remember, prevention starts with awareness. By learning to identify toxic behavior and setting clear boundaries, we can stop abuse before it begins—and create a future where everyone feels safe, respected, and valued in their relationships.

CHAPTER 9

LIFE AFTER ABUSE – RECLAIMING YOUR POWER

Leaving an emotionally and psychologically abusive relationship is one of the hardest things anyone can do. It takes an incredible amount of courage and strength to walk away from someone who has manipulated, controlled, and gaslighted you for months, or even years. However, once you've taken that step, the journey isn't over. In many ways, the real work begins after you leave.

For me, leaving was both a huge relief and a terrifying new chapter. I had spent so long trapped in my abuser's control that I wasn't sure who I was outside of the relationship. I had lost touch with my own identity, needs, and self-worth, and I had alienated those who could be a support system. But I knew that if I was going to heal, I had to start reclaiming my power. I had to rebuild my life from the ground up, rediscover who I was, and take back the control I had lost.

The journey of healing after abuse is long and often difficult. There are emotional ups and downs, moments of self-doubt, and days when it feels like you'll never fully recover. But there are also moments of incredible growth, strength, and self-discovery. Reclaiming your power after abuse isn't just about moving on—it's about learning to live life on your own terms again, without the shadow of your abuser hanging over you.

In this chapter, we'll explore the process of reclaiming your power after leaving an abusive relationship. We'll discuss the emotional ups and downs, the practical steps to rebuild your life, coping strategies for setbacks, and the importance of finding a new sense of purpose and identity. Additionally, we'll explore how sharing your story can empower both you and others.

The Healing Process: What to Expect After Leaving

When you first leave an emotionally and psychologically abusive relationship, you might expect to feel instant relief—and in many ways, you do. The weight of the constant manipulation, control, and fear is lifted, and you're finally free. But what many people don't realize is that the emotional rollercoaster often intensifies after leaving.

For me, the first few weeks after I left were a blur of emotions. I felt relieved, yes, but I also felt scared, confused, guilty, and deeply sad. I had spent so long in survival mode that I wasn't sure how to live without the constant tension and fear that had defined my life. It was as if my entire world had shifted, and I was left trying to figure out who I was without the person who had controlled so much of my life.

Here's what you can expect in the healing process after leaving:

1. **Relief and Fear**: The first emotion many survivors feel after leaving is relief. The constant tension, fear, and control are gone, and you're finally free to make your own choices again. But that relief is often accompanied by fear—fear of the unknown, fear of what comes next, and fear of the abuser trying to regain control. It's normal to feel both relieved and afraid at the same time.

2. **Anger and Sadness**: As the initial relief fades, many survivors experience a mix of anger and sadness. You might feel angry at your abuser for what they put you through, at yourself for not leaving sooner, or at the world for allowing this to happen. At the same time, you might feel deep sadness for the relationship you thought you had, for the time you lost, the money you lost, or for the person you used to be before the abuse.

3. **Confusion and Self-Doubt**: Emotional and psychological abuse often leaves survivors doubting

themselves and their perceptions. Even after leaving, it's common to second-guess your decision or wonder if you did the right thing. You might question whether the abuse was "really that bad," or whether you could have done something differently to make the relationship work. This confusion is a natural part of the healing process, but it's important to remind yourself that the abuse was real, and leaving was the right choice. You see this so often when it takes an average of seven times for someone to leave their abuser.

4. **Hope and Empowerment**: As you begin to heal, moments of hope and empowerment will start to emerge. You'll realize that you're stronger than you thought, that you have the power to rebuild your life, and that you deserve to be treated with love and respect. These moments of empowerment can be incredibly powerful, and they'll help carry you through the harder days.

In my own journey, these emotions didn't come in a linear order—they came in waves. Some days I felt strong and empowered; other days, I felt overwhelmed by shame, sadness, guilt, and self-doubt. But over time, the moments of strength became more frequent, and I began to see that life after abuse wasn't just about surviving—it was about thriving.

Rebuilding a Life of Independence and Self-Worth

One of the most important steps in reclaiming your power after abuse is rebuilding your life on your own terms. For so long, your decisions, actions, and even your thoughts were controlled by someone else. Now, it's time to take back that control and create a life that reflects your own needs, desires, and values.

Here are some practical steps you can take to rebuild your life after leaving an abusive relationship:

1. **Regaining Financial Independence**: Many survivors of abuse, especially those in financially controlling relationships, find themselves financially dependent on their abuser. Reclaiming your financial independence is critical to regaining control over your life. Start by assessing your financial situation, creating a budget, and taking steps to build your own financial security. This might mean finding a new job, opening a separate bank account, or seeking financial advice to help you get back on your feet.

   - **Tiffiny's Testimony**: For me, financial independence was one of the biggest hurdles after leaving. I had been so dependent on my abuser, he negatively impacted my ability to get a promotion or a pay increase at work, he manipulated me out of forty thousand dollars, I didn't know where to start. But once

I took control, educated myself on different aspects of finances, and changed careers, I felt like I was finally taking back control of my life. It wasn't easy, but it was one of the most empowering things I did in my recovery.

2. **Focusing on Personal Growth**: Rebuilding your life after abuse isn't just about practical steps—it's also about personal growth and self-discovery. Take time to explore your interests, hobbies, and passions. Reconnect with the things that make you feel alive and fulfilled. This could be anything from taking up a new hobby to pursuing further education or career development.

   ○ **Tiffiny's Testimony**: After I left my relationship, I realized how much of myself I had lost in the process. I had given up so many things that I loved—my hobbies, friendships, and sense of independence. Reconnecting with those things was a huge part of my healing journey.

3. **Building a Support System**: Healing from emotional and psychological abuse isn't something you have to do alone. Surround yourself with people who support you, believe in you, and uplift you. This might mean swallowing your pride and reaching out and reconnecting with old friends or family members, or it might mean finding new connections through support groups, therapy, or community organizations.

4. **Creating a Safe and Stable Environment**: One of the most important things you can do after leaving an abusive relationship is to create a safe and stable environment for yourself. This could mean finding a new place to live, establishing healthy routines, or creating a space that feels like your own. A stable environment can help you feel grounded and give you the foundation you need to rebuild your life.

Rebuilding your life after abuse is a process, and it's important to take things one step at a time. It's okay to start small—whether that's setting up a new bank account, taking up a hobby you love, or spending time with supportive friends. Each step you take is a step toward reclaiming your power and creating a life that reflects who you truly are.

How to Cope with Emotional Setbacks

Even after leaving an abusive relationship, emotional setbacks are inevitable. You might experience flashbacks, moments of self-doubt, or fear of entering new relationships. These setbacks can be difficult to deal with, but they're a normal part of the healing process.

Here are some strategies for coping with emotional setbacks:

1. **Recognize and Acknowledge Triggers**: Triggers are events, people, or situations that remind you of the

abuse and bring up painful emotions. It's important to recognize your triggers and understand that they're a natural response to trauma. When you experience a trigger, take a moment to acknowledge it and remind yourself that you're no longer in that abusive situation.

2. **Practice Self-Compassion**: After leaving an abusive relationship, it's common to struggle with self-doubt and feelings of guilt or shame. You might question whether you did the right thing or blame yourself for staying as long as you did. It's important to practice self-compassion during these moments. Remind yourself that the abuse wasn't your fault, and that you deserve kindness, love, and respect.

3. **Build Emotional Resilience**: Emotional resilience is the ability to bounce back from setbacks and continue moving forward. One way to build resilience is by practicing mindfulness and self-awareness. Pay attention to your thoughts and emotions, and learn to differentiate between healthy emotions and negative self-talk. When negative thoughts arise, challenge them with positive affirmations or reminders of your progress.

4. **Seek Professional Help**: If you're struggling with flashbacks, triggers, or emotional setbacks, it's important to seek professional help. A therapist can help you process the trauma and give you tools to cope with the emotional challenges that come with recovery.

Finding a New Purpose and Identity After Abuse

One of the most powerful steps in reclaiming your power after abuse is rediscovering your sense of purpose and identity. During the relationship, you may have lost touch with who you are outside of the abuse. Now, it's time to reconnect with yourself and define your own identity on your own terms.

Here's how to start finding a new sense of purpose and identity after abuse:

1. **Reconnect with Your Passions**: What are the things that make you feel alive? What are the hobbies, interests, or passions that you may have given up during the relationship? Take time to reconnect with the things that bring you joy and fulfillment. This might mean revisiting an old hobby, trying something new, or pursuing a passion that you've always wanted to explore.
   - **Tiffiny's Testimony**: After I left my relationship, I realized that I had lost touch with so many of the things I loved. I had stopped exploring, reading, volunteering, and spending time with people who made me feel good. Reconnecting with those passions was a huge part of my healing journey.
2. **Define Your Own Identity**: For so long, your identity may have been defined by your abuser—what they wanted, what they needed, and how they saw you.

Now, it's time to define your own identity on your terms. Reflect on who you are, what you value, and what you want out of life. Remember that you're not defined by the abuse—you're defined by the strength, resilience, and courage you've shown in overcoming it.

3. **Set New Goals**: One of the best ways to move forward after abuse is by setting new goals for yourself. These goals can be small or big—whether it's learning a new skill, pursuing a career, or building a new relationship. Setting goals gives you a sense of purpose and direction, helping you focus on the future rather than the past.

4. **Celebrate Your Progress**: As you begin to rebuild your life, it's essential to celebrate your progress. Whether it's taking a small step toward independence, overcoming a fear, or achieving a personal goal, acknowledging your progress can help you see how far you've come.

How Sharing Your Story Can Empower Others

One of the most empowering things you can do after surviving emotional and psychological abuse is to share your story. Sharing your experiences not only helps you heal, but it also helps break the silence around abuse and empowers others who may be going through similar situations.

Here's how sharing your story can empower both you and others:

1. **Breaking the Silence**: Emotional and psychological abuse thrives in silence. By sharing your story, you help break that silence and raise awareness about the realities and different types of abuse. You let others know that they're not alone, and that it's possible to survive and thrive after abuse.

2. **Empowering Yourself**: Sharing your story is a powerful way to take control of your own narrative. It allows you to reflect on your experiences, acknowledge your strength, and celebrate your resilience. By owning your story, you take back the power that was taken from you during the relationship.

3. **Inspiring Others**: Your story has the power to inspire others who may be in similar situations. By sharing your experiences, you give hope to others who may feel trapped or powerless. You show them that it's possible to leave, to heal, and to rebuild a life after abuse.

   o **Tiffiny's Testimony**: When I started sharing my story, I was amazed at how many people reached out to me to say that they had been through something similar. Sharing my experiences not only helped me heal, but it also helped others see that they weren't alone.

4. **Practical Tips for Sharing Your Story**: If you're ready to share your story, start by finding a safe and supportive space. This could be through a support group, a blog, or even a close group of friends. Remember that sharing your story is a personal

decision, and you don't have to share everything if you're not ready. Start small, and only share what feels comfortable to you.

Conclusion: Reclaiming Your Power, One Step at a Time

Reclaiming your power after emotional and psychological abuse is a journey, but it's a journey worth taking. It's about rediscovering who you are, rebuilding your life on your own terms, and finding a new sense of purpose and identity. It's about healing from the pain of the past and moving forward with strength, resilience, and hope.

Remember that this process takes time, and it's okay to take things one step at a time. You've already shown incredible strength by leaving the abuse, and now it's time to continue that journey of healing and empowerment. Reclaim your power, one step at a time, and know that you are capable of creating a life that is filled with love, respect, and self-worth.

CHAPTER 10

BREAKING THE SILENCE AROUND EMOTIONAL ABUSE

Emotional and psychological abuse is a form of control that thrives in silence. Unlike physical abuse, which often leaves visible scars, emotional and psychological abuse is insidious—it's hidden behind closed doors, masked by smiles, and cloaked in secrecy. For many survivors, admitting that they are being emotionally abused is one of the hardest things they will ever do. The fear of judgment, guilt, shame, and not being believed keeps them locked in silence.

This silence does more than just protect the abuser—it allows the abuse to continue unchecked. When no one talks about emotional and psychological abuse, it becomes easier for abusers to manipulate their victims without fear of consequence. The silence also makes it harder for victims/survivors to recognize what's happening to them, leaving them feeling isolated, confused, and alone.

For me, breaking the silence was the first step toward reclaiming my voice and my power. For years, I had convinced myself that what I was experiencing wasn't "real" abuse, because there were no physical scars. I told myself that I was just overreacting, that my partner's behavior wasn't that bad. But deep down, I knew something was wrong. It wasn't until I started talking about my experiences—first with a therapist, and eventually with others who had been through similar situations—that I realized just how much damage had been done.

Speaking out wasn't easy. I was ashamed that I had allowed myself to get into this situation, and guilt for allowing it to continue for so long. But the more I shared my story, the more I realized that I wasn't alone. With every conversation, I felt a little bit stronger, a little bit more empowered. Breaking the silence didn't just help me heal—it helped others understand that emotional abuse is real, and it's just as damaging as any other form of abuse.

Abusers thrive in secrecy; they rely on societal misconceptions about what abuse looks like. Knowing that without visible bruises or broken bones, their actions may go unnoticed or dismissed, they continue their manipulation.

Throughout my relationship, I was made to believe that everything that went wrong was my fault. If I didn't follow the rules—about how I dressed, who I spoke to, or even what I posted on social media—there were consequences. If I didn't behave the way he wanted, he would withdraw affection, leaving me feeling worthless and desperate for his approval.

The coercive control even extended into how he would manipulate others' perceptions of me. When I discovered he had signed up for Ashley Madison on my birthday, he not only denied it but twisted the narrative so that I was the unreasonable one. This tactic, known as DARVO (Deny, Attack, and Reverse Victim and Offender), left me doubting my reality, questioning if I was overreacting or making things up.

Breaking the silence means sharing these stories—stories of gaslighting, manipulation, and the deep psychological wounds that they leave. It's about empowering others to see the signs early and take action to protect themselves and their loved ones.

This chapter is about breaking that silence, not just for survivors but for everyone. It's about creating a culture where emotional abuse is no longer hidden or dismissed, where people feel safe to talk about their experiences without fear of judgment. It's about empowering survivors to find their voices, and encouraging friends, family, and communities to play an active role in supporting those affected by emotional abuse.

Creating Safe Spaces for Open Dialogue

One of the most important steps in breaking the silence around emotional abuse is creating safe spaces for sharing their experiences. Emotional abuse often leaves survivors feeling isolated, ashamed, and guilty, making it difficult for them to reach out for help. By fostering environments of trust and non-judgmental support, we can create spaces where survivors feel seen, heard, and understood.

So how do we create these safe spaces? Here are some practical steps:

1. **Fostering Trust**: Trust is the foundation of any safe space. Whether in a family, friendship, or a community group, people need to feel that they can trust those around them to listen without judgment. This means being patient, compassionate, and respecting their boundaries and confidentiality.
   - **Tiffiny's Testimony**: I remember the first time I told a friend about what I was going through. I was so full of shame and guilt, scared she wouldn't believe the extent. But instead, she listened without trying to fix the situation. That moment made all the difference; it showed me that I wasn't alone, and that people cared.

2. **Encouraging Open Conversations**: Emotional abuse thrives in secrecy. We must create an environment where open conversations are encouraged, discussing healthy relationships, boundaries, and emotional well-being in your family and community. No topic is off-limits, and people can discuss their experiences without fear of judgment or dismissal.

3. **Offering Support Without Pressure**: Survivors of emotional abuse often feel immense pressure to make decisions about their relationship—whether that's to stay, leave, or confront their abuser. In a safe space, the goal is to offer support without adding to that pressure. Let them know that you're there for them no matter what they decide, and that you'll support them at their own pace.

4. **Normalizing Discussions About Mental Health**: Emotional and psychological abuse can take a serious toll on mental health, leading to anxiety, depression, and developing physical issues. By normalizing discussions about mental health and seeking help, we create a culture where people feel comfortable talking about their emotional well-being without stigma.

Creating safe spaces is essential for helping survivors of emotional abuse find their voice. When people feel safe to talk about their experiences, they begin to reclaim their power and take steps toward healing.

How Friends, Family, and Communities Can Help Break the Silence

Emotional abuse doesn't just affect the person experiencing it—it affects everyone around them. It's like a tornado. Friends, family members, and communities have a crucial role to play in breaking the silence and supporting survivors. Unfortunately, many people don't know how to recognize emotional or psychological abuse, or they don't know how to help someone who is going through it.

Here's how you can help break the silence and support someone who is experiencing emotional abuse:

1. **Recognizing the Signs of Emotional Abuse**: Educate yourself about the signs which can include constant criticism, manipulation, isolation, gaslighting, and controlling behavior. If you notice these signs in someone's relationship, don't ignore them. Approach the situation with care and concern, and let the person know that you're there for them if they need support.

    o **Tiffiny's Testimony**: For a long time, I didn't even realize I was being emotionally abused. It wasn't until a close work friend gently pointed out some of the red flags in a story I shared with her, helping me see things clearly. Her willingness to talk to me about it—even though it was a difficult conversation—made all the difference.

2. **Being a Supportive Listener**: Listen without judgment or trying to "fix" the situation. Survivors often feel shame or guilt about their situation, and they need to know that they aren't being judged for staying in the relationship or for not leaving sooner. Offer a listening ear, validate their feelings, and let them know that they're not alone.

   ○ **What to say**: "I'm really sorry you're going through this, and I'm here for you whenever you need to talk. You deserve to be treated with respect and kindness."

   ○ **What not to say**: "Why don't you just leave?" or "I would never let someone treat me that way." These kinds of statements can deepen feelings of isolation and shame.

3. **Offering Practical Help**: Survivors often feel trapped and powerless. Offering practical help—whether helping them find resources, connecting them with a therapist, or even just being there for them during a difficult moment—can make a huge difference. Let them know that you're there to support them in whatever way they need, whether that's emotional support or practical assistance.

4. **Respecting Their Boundaries**: It's crucial to respect the survivor's boundaries. Leaving an abusive relationship is a deeply personal decision, and it often takes

time. Pushing someone to leave before they're ready can make them feel even more isolated or confused. These confused feelings often have them returning to the abuser. Instead, offer support and let them know that you'll be there for them no matter what they decide.

5. **Challenging Harmful Attitudes in Your Community**: Breaking the silence around emotional and psychological abuse requires challenging harmful attitudes and beliefs in our communities. This includes speaking out against victim-blaming, calling out abusive behavior when we see it, and educating others about what emotional abuse looks like. By raising awareness and challenging harmful norms, we can create a culture where abuse is no longer tolerated or hidden.

Challenging Cultural Norms That Perpetuate Emotional Abuse

Emotional abuse doesn't happen in a vacuum—it's often perpetuated by cultural norms and societal beliefs that normalize control, manipulation, and unhealthy power dynamics in relationships. These norms can make it difficult for survivors to recognize their situations, and can also discourage people from speaking out against abuse.

One of the most common cultural norms that perpetuates emotional abuse is the belief that jealousy and possessiveness are signs of love or care. Many people, especially women, are taught that controlling actions are signs that their partner "cares too much." In reality, these behaviors are red flags for emotional abuse.

Here are some other cultural norms that perpetuate emotional abuse, and how we can challenge them:

1. **Gender Stereotypes**: Traditional gender roles and stereotypes contribute to emotional abuse. For example, men are often taught to be dominant and controlling in relationships, while women are expected to be submissive and accommodating. These power dynamics can create an environment where emotional abuse is normalized, and where victims feel like they have to stay silent to meet societal expectations.

    o **Challenging Gender Norms**: We can challenge these stereotypes by promoting equality and mutual respect in relationships. This means encouraging open communication, shared decision-making, and equal power dynamics between partners. It also means raising awareness about the ways in which traditional gender roles can contribute to emotional abuse. We all have a voice.

2. **Cultural Expectations of Silence**: In many cultures, there is an expectation that personal or family matters should be kept private. This can make it hard for survivors of emotional abuse to speak out, especially

if they fear that they'll bring shame or dishonor to their family. These cultural expectations of silence can create an environment where abuse goes unspoken and unaddressed.

    ○ **Encouraging Open Conversations**: We can challenge these cultural expectations by encouraging open conversations about emotional well-being and healthy relationships. This means breaking down the stigma around abuse and creating spaces where people feel comfortable talking about their experiences without fear of judgment or shame.

3. **Normalization of Toxic Behavior in Media**: Emotional and psychological abuse is often normalized in the media, whether it's through movies, TV shows, or music. Toxic behaviors like jealousy, manipulation, coercion or control are sometimes romanticized or portrayed as signs of passion. This can make it harder for people to recognize emotional abuse in their own relationships, especially if they've seen and internalized these messages from a young age.

    ○ **Promoting Healthy Representations**: We can challenge the normalization of emotional and psychological abuse in the media by promoting healthy representations of relationships. This means supporting media that portrays relationships based on respect, communication, and equality, and calling out media that romanticizes toxic behavior and teaching our children the difference.

By challenging these cultural norms, we create a society where emotional abuse is no longer tolerated or minimized. It starts with raising awareness, having open conversations, and promoting healthy relationships in our families, communities, and media.

Raising Awareness and Educating Others About Emotional Abuse

Raising awareness about emotional and psychological abuse is one of the most powerful ways to break the silence and prevent abuse from happening in the future. The more people understand emotional abuse, the more likely they are to recognize it in their own lives or the lives of others.

Here are some ways you can raise awareness and educate others about emotional abuse:

1. **Sharing Your Story**: One of the most effective ways to raise awareness about emotional abuse is by sharing your experiences. When survivors speak out, it not only highlights the realities of emotional abuse and the damage it can cause. It also encourages other survivors to come forward and share their own stories, creating a ripple effect of awareness and empowerment.

- ○ **Tiffiny's Testimony**: Sharing my story was one of the scariest things I've ever done, yet it was also one of the most empowering. I realized that by speaking out, I was helping others see that they weren't alone–that emotional and psychological abuse, like all forms of abuse, is real and valid.

2. **Educating Others About the Signs of Emotional Abuse**: Many people struggle to recognize emotional abuse, especially if they've never experienced it themselves. By informing others about the signs of emotional abuse—such as manipulation, gaslighting, isolation, and control—you empower them to identify these red flags in their own lives or those of people they care about.

3. **Using Social Media to Spread Awareness**: Social media is a powerful tool for spreading awareness about emotional and psychological abuse. By sharing articles, resources, and personal stories across social media platforms, you can reach a wide audience, helping to educate others about the harsh realities of emotional abuse. Additionally, social media allows for connection with others who are committed to raising awareness and supporting survivors.

4. **Supporting Organizations That Work to Prevent Emotional Abuse**: Numerous organizations work tirelessly to prevent domestic abuse and support survivors. By contributing through donations,

volunteering, or spreading awareness—you can play a role in their essential work.

Empowering Loved Ones to Break Free from Abuse and Find Their Voices

One of the most vital roles you can play in breaking the silence around emotional abuse is to empower your loved ones to find their voices. Whether they remain in an abusive relationship or have already left, survivors often struggle with feelings of shame, guilt, and self-doubt. Your support and encouragement can help them reclaim their power and find the confidence to speak out.

Here's how you can empower your loved ones to break free from abuse and find their voices:

1. **Encourage Open Dialogue**: One of the most transformative steps for a survivor is to speak out. Encourage your loved one to share their experiences in a way that feels safe and empowering–whether with a therapist, a support group, or even close friends. Remind them that their story matters, and that speaking out can be a powerful tool for healing.

2. **Validate Their Experience**: Emotional abuse can leave survivors questioning their own experiences and doubting their perceptions. By affirming their feelings and experiences, you help them rebuild their confidence and trust in themselves. Let them know that

what they went through was real, and that they deserve to be heard.

3. **Help Them Set Boundaries**: Reclaiming one's voice involves learning to set boundaries and assert your needs. Support your loved one in practicing boundary-setting within their relationships, whether with friends, family members, or new partners. Encourage them to prioritize their own emotional well-being and to speak up when something doesn't feel right.

4. **Celebrating Their Progress**: Healing from emotional abuse is a journey that requires acknowledgement of small victories. Whether it's speaking out for the first time, establishing a boundary, or taking steps toward independence, celebrate these milestones and let your loved one know how proud you are of their progress. t

A Collective Call to Action

Breaking the silence around emotional abuse isn't just the responsibility of survivors—it's a collective call to action for all of us. Whether you're a friend, a family member, or a community leader, you have the power to raise awareness, create safe spaces, and support those affected by emotional abuse.

By speaking out, educating others, and challenging harmful cultural norms, we can create a world where emotional and psychological abuse is no longer hidden in the shadows. Together, we can empower survivors to find their voices, reclaim their power, and live lives free from control and manipulation.

Let's break the silence together.

CHAPTER 11

A JOURNEY THROUGH THE DARKNESS - TIFFINY'S STORY

As we conclude our exploration of emotional and psychological abuse, I invite you to step into my personal journey. What follows is a deeply personal, novel-style account of my own experience with domestic abuse, the subtle and overt ways it infiltrated my life, and the difficult yet empowering process of healing and reclaiming my sense of self. This narrative is raw, honest, and at times painful to read, but it serves an essential purpose: to show how the red flags, cycles, and patterns we've discussed throughout this book come to life in the everyday experience of abuse. As you read, you'll see how emotional manipulation, isolation, and control can gradually escalate into more severe forms of abuse. You'll also witness the slow realization of what's happening, the struggle to escape, and the ongoing process of healing. My hope is that by sharing my story, you will gain a deeper understanding of how emotional and psychological abuse can take hold and the strength it takes to break free, empowering you to recognize and confront it in your life or the lives of those you love.

The Beginning – December 2016: Meeting Him

I met him at the dog park across from my apartment in Channelside, Tampa, in December 2016. It felt serendipitous, like we were meant to meet. We talked for hours, and I remember thinking, *Where has this guy been?* He was charming, attentive, and seemed genuinely interested in everything I had to say. We didn't even exchange numbers, but that encounter left a lasting impression.

I spent Christmas with my family, then flew to Australia by myself for New Year's, feeling empowered and independent. Life was good. I had no idea that the man from the dog park was about to come back into my life and change everything.

January 2017: The Reconnection

When I returned from Australia, life returned to its normal rhythm—until one day, I saw him again at the dog park. It felt like fate was giving me a second chance. This time, we exchanged numbers and went on a date. Things moved quickly after that. He lived in the condo building across the street, which made it easy for us to spend time together. We were practically inseparable. Gym dates, dinners, movies—everything seemed perfect.

He seemed to share my values about loyalty, and we talked about how neither of us wanted drama in our lives. I believed him. When I fell asleep in his arms, I felt secure, like I had finally found someone who understood me. But looking back, that feeling of security was just the start of his control.

February 2017: Subtle Manipulation Begins

The first signs of trouble came in February. I needed a night to organize documents for an important meeting with my accountant, so I told him I couldn't spend the night. Instead of understanding, he took it personally. He said my decision made him feel "worthless." It seemed like an overreaction, but I didn't think much of it at the time. I brushed it off, thinking I was just misreading his reaction.

Looking back, I see this moment as a red flag. It was the first time he used emotional manipulation to make me feel guilty for having my own needs. He later used that night against me, planting the seed of doubt in my mind about my priorities.

Valentine's Day came, and he showered me with gifts—a sapphire and white gold bracelet—and we took a romantic trip to Miami. It was supposed to be perfect. But looking back, even then, something felt off. At dinner, despite my happiness, he leaned in and said, "You don't seem excited to be here." That comment stung. I had been smiling, feeling content, yet somehow, it wasn't enough for him. That was the start of his grooming pattern: no matter what I did, he always found a way to make me feel like I wasn't doing enough.

March 2017: Isolation and Control Begin

In March, things started to escalate. He bought a condo on Clearwater Beach and invited me to help with the design, making it seem like he wanted to build a future together. It felt like a commitment, but what I didn't realize at the time was that this 'future casting' was another way to control me, to make me feel more invested and dependent on him.

His control over my social life began soon after. He scrutinized my Facebook, questioning why I hadn't updated my relationship status. He didn't like that I had male friends or even certain female friends, and he insisted I remove them from my social media. "They aren't good for us," he'd say. I started deleting people to avoid fights, slowly cutting myself off from friends. I was losing my support system, and he was becoming my whole world.

April 2017: The Witch Hunt

By April, his control over me deepened. He demanded access to my phone, email, and social media accounts, claiming that if I had nothing to hide, I should have no problem sharing everything. I wasn't hiding anything, so I gave him my passwords, hoping it would calm his insecurities. But instead, it became a way for him to dig deeper into my past, scrutinizing every message, every interaction.

He found old emails from ex-boyfriends, and even though they were years old, he demanded I delete entire email accounts to erase any trace of them. He went through my Facebook photos, finding pictures with male friends and accusing me of things that had never happened. His paranoia was suffocating, and I complied with his demands because it was easier than fighting. Every day became a new test of my loyalty, and I was failing by his standards.

May-June 2017: The Entitlement and Sexual Control

By the time summer came, he felt entitled to control not just my life but my body. He expected sex on his terms—every morning before the gym. If I resisted or wasn't enthusiastic enough, it led to fights. He started controlling my physical appearance too, dictating what I wore to work and how I dressed around him. If I wore heels to work but not around him, he accused me of trying to impress other men.

One day at the gym, a friend came over to say hello, and afterward, he berated me, saying I shouldn't be friends with someone who "rudely interrupted" our time. He started creating barriers between me and my friends, isolating me further. He wanted to be the only one in my life.

The sexual demands became a regular part of our relationship. If I didn't comply, there were consequences. It was easier to give in than to face the inevitable fights and punishment that followed.

July-August 2017: Physical Violence Begins

July was when the abuse turned physical. We were in Panama City on what was supposed to be a fun getaway, but it quickly turned into another nightmare. A simple text from a friend's husband about work sparked his jealousy, and he started a fight, accusing me of having feelings for the man. The argument escalated, and before I knew it, he had grabbed me, pushing me against the wall.

That was the first time he physically hurt me, and I was in shock. I didn't want to believe it was real. I thought it was a one-time thing, that maybe I had done something to provoke him. But it wasn't a one-time thing. It was the beginning of another level of control.

After that, the violence became more frequent. If I didn't meet his expectations—whether it was about sex, my appearance, or how I interacted with other people—he lashed out. Sometimes it was physical, but most often it was coercion, chipping away at my self-esteem, making me feel like I was always in the wrong.

September 2017: Humiliation and Betrayal

September brought more betrayal. We celebrated my birthday with a family dinner, and though the evening went well, it ended with him berating me for not initiating a birthday photo with him. By the time we got home, I was in tears. He had an uncanny ability to ruin even the most joyous moments.

Later that month, I discovered he had signed up for Ashley Madison—the day before my birthday. He denied it, blaming it on a contractor, but I knew better. This is when I started documenting everything. I had been walking on eggshells, trying to keep him happy, only to find out he had been betraying me all along. I wanted to make sure I wasn't 'seeing things'.

October-November 2017: The Presentation and Continued Manipulation

By October, I had moved out of my own apartment and essentially lived in his condo. My lease was up, and I mentioned moving in together officially. He told me I had to put together a presentation to explain why it would be a good idea. At first, I thought he was joking, but he wasn't. It was just another way for him to assert his control and belittle me.

He continued his emotional manipulation, accusing me of not doing enough for him while using my financial resources.

I cashed out $40,000 from my retirement account to help him recast the mortgage on his condo, thinking it was for our future. But after every argument, he made it clear that I was just a "guest" in his home. He constantly reminded me of my supposed inadequacies, using guilt to control me financially and emotionally.

December 2017: The Holidays Ruined

The holidays, which should have been a time of joy, were filled with tension. We made Christmas ornaments from sand dollars we had collected on the beach, decorated a beautiful tree, and even attended a concert at his church. But a simple compliment I gave about the singer turned into a massive fight. He accused me of ruining the evening, and after that, we never went back to church together. It was another reminder that nothing I did was ever enough for him.

January-March 2018: Spy Cameras and Deeper Control

By January 2018, the relationship had reached a new low. I discovered a hidden camera in the clock by the bed, placed there to spy on me. When I confronted him, he exploded, accusing me of being paranoid and turning the blame on me. He was monitoring my every move, even when I was asleep. I was no longer just emotionally trapped—I was physically surveilled.

In February, his control over our sex life became even more pronounced. He would go weeks without touching me, claiming I didn't deserve affection because I wasn't attractive enough or wasn't doing what he wanted. Yet, he still expected me to perform sexual acts for him on demand. If I didn't comply, he would threaten to find someone else who would.

April-May 2018: The Physical Abuse Intensifies

The physical abuse intensified in April and May. We had a massive argument after meeting him at the airport, and he accused me of disrespecting him. He screamed and yelled at me while I was driving to the level I had to stop the car. I asked him to get out. He took my purse and dropped it in the middle of the road as he walked away. When I got back to the condo, he grabbed me, shoved me, and punched me in the chest. He took my keys and threw me out of the condo with my dog. I was stranded, humiliated, and scared. Later that night, he cheated on me, calling a woman he had previously blocked on my social media.

The next day, he begged me to come back, saying he loved me, but I knew it was just another manipulation. He wanted me back under his control.

Summer 2018: Reaching Out for Therapy

By mid-2018, I knew something had to change, but I still felt trapped. I began to question my own sanity, wondering if I was the problem. In an effort to find clarity, I reached out to an online therapy service called BetterHelp. I didn't tell him. Therapy became my secret lifeline.

During my sessions, the therapist pointed out the patterns of emotional and psychological abuse I had been enduring. I was still in denial at first, convinced that if I could just "fix" myself, the relationship would improve. But with each session, I began to see the truth: I wasn't the problem. He was.

The therapist helped me understand the cycle of abuse I was caught in—the love-bombing, the isolation, the manipulation, and the escalating violence. I finally saw how deeply he had eroded my sense of self-worth, how he had twisted my reality to make me doubt my every thought and action. Therapy was my first real step toward reclaiming my life.

June-September 2018: The Plan to Escape

By summer 2018, I had started quietly planning my escape. I already had a storage unit, from my condo move, and began stashing away my belongings and building up a 'to go bag', bit by bit. I knew I couldn't leave suddenly. He would have made sure

I had nowhere to go. But I had to get out before the situation escalated even further.

I continued to endure his emotional abuse, his guilt demands for money, and his constant surveillance. But I knew that I was reaching a breaking point. I was preparing to leave, even if it meant starting over with nothing.

Especially after being sent 'The List'

THE LIST

Nonstarters for me to continue and most importantly for us to have a loving relationship that lasts. I need to see these happen immediately. Some had happened but have stopped. When I see this is done completely and out of love, I will be open to possible changes. *Read and memorize the list so it's never again a question of 'not knowing'.*

1. No Social media other than FB
2. We are the focus of FB to show everyone how happy you are with me
3. You will post frequently about me/us
4. You will like/comment my posts
5. People I don't approve won't be on there due to past bs
6. You will tell me in person by voice of any changes messages texts on your phone
7. You will ask to play on your personal phone at home

8. Your phone will be put on silent at 7 pm with exceptions for favorites
9. You will not move or cover security cameras making them always visible
10. You won't go outside alone
11. You will go to condo gym only when I'm gone, and only prior to work
12. You will tell me when you arrive and leave work, and notify me of any exceptions
13. You will look to me as the leader
14. You will give as much as you possibly can in terms of deeds, acts of service, and financial obligations.
15. I will manage the finances
16. I expect to be greeted at the airport
17. You will no longer interrupt me in front of co workers
18. You will no longer interrupt me in front of my mother
19. You will no longer disagree with me in front of others
20. You will look to me for guidance and accept my advice
21. You will say good morning and goodnight with happiness at a sound level in which I can hear. If you hear nothing in return it means I didn't hear it so repeat it.
22. You will listen when I'm talking
23. You will not cuss at me
24. You will not infer I'm not manly
25. You will wear what I like around the house and to bed
26. You will wear heels or dresses/sexy attire nightly/daily for sex without me having to ask. If you do not have what I like I'll take you shopping.

27. You will listen to what/how I want sex and learn.
28. You will stop moaning and groaning like you're old to move in bed. I need variety but cant do it if you cannot move. I need you to be your flexible self (like in the gym) and move faster.
29. You will quit talking to dogs when you are wanting to please me.
30. You will refrain from watching firemen take off theirs shirts and watching on tv
31. You will compliment me as young looking, good looking, and lucky to have.
32. You will ask prior to scheduling appointments
33. You will discuss in person anything you receive on your phone unless a delivery or parents. We will delete together.
34. You will always give me full access to stuff, and will tell me immediately if you have to change a password
35. You will get in the best shape physically for me
36. You will eat properly, and assist me as well
37. You will speak your mind and thoughts with the right respectful calm approach that shows me the respect I deserve
38. You will walk in front or beside me
39. Unless I can't I will open doors
40. You will appreciate what I have done and do for you
41. You will stick up for me, defending me at all times

October 2018: The Final Breaking Point

The final breaking point came in October 2018. I was working from home, taking phone calls for my job, when he walked into the room, dropped his pants, and demanded that I give him a blowjob. When I refused, he coldly said, "If you don't give me the sex I need, I'll find someone who will."

In that moment, I knew I had to leave. I packed my things, grabbed my dog, and walked out of the condo for the last time. I didn't look back. That night, I stayed in a hotel, and though I felt scared and uncertain, I also felt something I hadn't felt in years—freedom.

The Aftermath: Breaking Free

Even after I left, he continued to try to manipulate me—sending emails, making promises to change, begging me to come back. But I knew better. I had finally seen through the lies. The cycle of abuse—emotional, physical, financial, religious and psychological—was clear to me now. He had isolated me from my friends, taken control of my finances, and manipulated me into doubting myself at every turn.

But I was free. It took almost two years, but I had finally broken the cycle.

The Cycle of Abuse: Recognizing the Red Flags

Looking back, the cycle of abuse and the red flags were there from the beginning. The subtle manipulation, the isolation, the control over my body and my life. Abuse doesn't always start with a punch or a slap. Sometimes it starts with a comment, a subtle shift in power, a quiet erosion of your sense of self. But now, I can see it for what it was.

Leaving wasn't easy, and healing is an ongoing process. But I've reclaimed my life, and I'm learning to trust myself again. Abuse doesn't define me—survival does.

Today: A Warrior For Change

Six years have passed since I walked out of his condo, terrified yet determined. Looking back, I barely recognize the woman I was then. The journey has been challenging, but it has transformed me in ways I never could have imagined.

Today, I stand not just as a survivor, but as a warrior for change. My pain has become my purpose, my trauma has been transformed into a fierce drive to empower others. As an independent life insurance broker, I help women secure their financial futures. Through my business consulting company, NewTide Consulting LLC, I guide others in building their dreams on solid foundations. Yet, it's my role as President and co-founder of the IgniteHer, INC, 501c3. that truly ignites my passion. Here, I have the privilege of supporting women through their own journeys of healing and self-discovery.

The path to healing has been long and, at times, grueling. Countless hours of counseling, deep introspection, and hard work have helped me recognize and change toxic patterns. With each step forward, I reclaim a piece of myself. My journey led me to Gracie Jiu-Jitsu Largo, where I am pursuing certification to teach self defense through their Women Empowered program. There's profound satisfaction in equipping women with the skills to protect themselves and stand strong in their power.

I've immersed myself in understanding the complexities of domestic violence, attending conferences like the FL Domestic Violence Coalition Conference and the Training Institute on Strangulation Prevention. These experiences have deepened my resolve to make a difference. I actively participate in local Sexual Assault Response Team and Domestic Violence Task Force meetings, always seeking new ways to support victims, survivors, and fellow advocates.

One of the most healing aspects of my journey has been reconnecting with the relationships that were severed during my time with DBS. Rebuilding these bonds has reminded me of the strength found in genuine connections. I now share my story widely now, no longer bound by shame or fear. Every time I speak, I hope to plant seeds of recognition, helping others identify the early signs of abuse that I once missed. I focus on safe exit strategies and preventive measures, determined that others should not endure what I did.

Looking to the future, my mission is clear: to empower women to recognize their worth, to harness their stories as superpowers, and to access the courage that has always resided within them. Through a blend of self-defense training, mindfulness yoga, and strategic education, I'm collaborating with various organizations to provide comprehensive resources for women. My goal is to help them build independent, safe, and fulfilling lives.

As I stand here today, I am living proof that there is life after abuse – a rich, purposeful, joyous life. From the ashes of my past, I have risen like a phoenix, stronger and more radiant than before. My scars are no longer sources of shame, they are badges of honor, testaments to my resilience.

To anyone out there who might be where I once was, know this: you are stronger than you know. Your story isn't over; it's just beginning. There's a whole community of survivors ready to support you when you're ready to take that first step.

As for me, my journey continues. Every woman I help, every story I share, every life I touch – these are the true measures of my healing. In helping others find their strength, I continuously rediscover my own.

This is not the end of my story; it's a new chapter, filled with purpose, hope, and an unwavering commitment to creating a world where every woman can live free from fear, embracing her full potential.

The girl who once stood in that dog park, unaware of the trials ahead, could never have imagined this future. But here I am, living proof that from the deepest darkness can come the most brilliant light.

This is my story. This is my truth. And I am no longer afraid to shine.

A Call to Action: Advocating for Change and Supporting Survivors

The journey of healing from emotional and psychological abuse is long and often fraught with pain and uncertainty, but it is a journey worth taking. Whether you are a survivor, a loved one of someone who has endured abuse, or an ally who wants to advocate for change, we must all unite to break the cycle of abuse, raise awareness, and create a culture of empathy and support.

When I began writing this book, my goal was to shed light on the hidden, often unspoken aspects of emotional and psychological abuse. As a survivor, I understand how insidious this type of abuse can be, and I recognize the vital importance of speaking out and taking action. The abuse I endured may not have left visible scars, but the wounds it inflicted were deep and lasting. It took time to heal, but I realized that healing wasn't just about moving on from the past—it was about taking back control of my life and using my voice to make a difference.

This final chapter is a call to action. Awareness is the first step, but it is not enough on its own. We must actively participate in creating a world where emotional and psychological abuse is no longer tolerated, where survivors are supported, and where future generations can live free from manipulation and control. It's time to transform everything we've learned into action— whether in our personal lives, within our communities, or across society at large.

Summarizing Key Lessons from the Book

As we bring this book to a close, it's crucial to reflect on the key lessons we've explored. Emotional and psychological abuse is complex, but understanding it is the first step toward healing and prevention. Let's recap some of the most important takeaways:

1. **Recognizing the Signs of Emotional and Psychological Abuse**: Abuse doesn't always leave physical scars, yet its effects are just as damaging. Emotional abuse can take many forms, including manipulation, gaslighting, isolation, control, and constant criticism. Early recognition of these signs, both in your own

relationships and in the lives of those around you. Understanding the red flags is vital for taking action before the abuse escalates into something physical.

2. **Supporting Loved Ones in Abusive Relationships**: When someone you care about is in an abusive relationship, your instinct might be to tell them to leave or to fix the situation. However, leaving an abusive relationship is a deeply personal decision that often takes time. The best way to support you is non-judgmental support, listening to their needs, and empowering them to make their own decisions.

3. **Rebuilding Self-Worth and Setting Boundaries**: After leaving an abusive relationship, a crucial step in healing is rebuilding your sense of self-worth. Abusers often erode their victims' confidence and make them feel powerless, but reclaiming your power is possible. Establishing healthy boundaries, prioritizing your own emotional well-being, and surrounding yourself with supportive people are all essential steps in the recovery process.

4. **Breaking the Silence Around Emotional Abuse**: Emotional abuse thrives in silence. By sharing your experiences, you not only initiate your own healing, but also raise awareness and help others recognize the signs of abuse. Whether you're a survivor, a friend, or an ally, breaking the silence is a powerful way to challenge the stigma around emotional abuse and foster change in your community.

These lessons form the foundation of this book, equipping you with the tools needed to advocate for yourself and others. But these lessons are just the beginning—what matters most is what you choose to do with this knowledge.

How You Can Make a Difference in the Lives of Survivors

One of the most impactful ways you can make a difference is by supporting the survivors in your life. Whether it's a friend, family member, colleague, or community member, your role as a supportive and empathetic presence can significantly impact their healing journey. Survivors often feel alone, misunderstood, or judged, but you have the power to change that.

Here's how you can help:

1. **Listen Without Judgment**: Survivors need compassionate listeners who won't try to "fix" the situation or pass judgment. Validate their feelings and reassure them that what they experienced is real and deserves to be heard.
   - **What to say**: "I believe you. What you went through is valid, and you didn't deserve any of it."
   - **What not to say**: "Why didn't you leave sooner?" or "You should have known better."

These statements only reinforce the survivor's feelings of guilt and shame.

2. **Offer Practical Support**: Survivors may need practical help—whether it's connecting them with resources, helping them find therapy, or even assisting with legal matters. Offer to research options, find community support groups, or attend appointments with them if they feel comfortable.

3. **Empower Them to Make Their Own Decisions**: Emotional abuse strips victims of autonomy and control. It's crucial to empower survivors to make their own choices about how to move forward. Avoid pushing them to take certain actions—whether that's leaving the relationship, confronting the abuser, or seeking legal action—until they're ready.

4. **Encourage Self-Compassion and Healing**: Survivors often struggle with feelings of shame, guilt, and self-blame. Encourage them to practice self-compassion and remind them that healing is a gradual process. Let them know that it's okay to take small steps and that recovery isn't linear.

   o **Tiffiny's Testimony**: For me, one of the most powerful parts of my healing journey was learning to be kind to myself. After years of feeling inadequate, rebuilding my confidence took time. Having people in my life who encouraged me to be gentle with myself made all the difference.

The Role of Communities in Preventing Emotional and Psychological Abuse

Communities play a vital role in preventing emotional and psychological abuse. Whether in schools, workplaces, religious institutions, or local organizations, creating environments where abuse is recognized, addressed, and prevented can have a profound impact on individuals and families.

Here are some ways communities can actively work to prevent emotional abuse:

1. **Creating Supportive Environments**: Promote open conversations about emotional well-being, healthy relationships, and mental health. When people feel supported and understood, they're more likely to speak out about abuse and seek help when needed.

    o **Schools and Educational Institutions**: Schools can educate students about healthy relationships, consent, and emotional intelligence from a young age. Integrating lessons on empathy, boundaries, and communication into the curriculum empowers the next generation to build respectful relationships.

    o **Workplaces**: Implement policies addressing emotional abuse, harassment, and toxic behavior in professional settings. Employers can offer resources like counseling services and employee support programs to ensure that staff have access to necessary support.

2. **Raising Awareness Through Community Initiatives**: Community organizations can play a crucial role in raising awareness about emotional abuse. Workshops, support groups, or public awareness campaigns, local organizations can educate people about the signs of emotional abuse and offer resources for survivors.

3. **Challenging Harmful Cultural Norms**: Communities must actively challenge cultural norms that minimize or dismiss emotional abuse. Whether it's addressing toxic masculinity, or rigid gender roles, efforts to dismantle these beliefs can foster a healthier environment. This can be achieved through public education campaigns and advocating for inclusive policies.

   o **Tiffiny's Testimony**: Looking back, I accepted many behaviors from my abuser, thinking they were just part of being in a relationship. After escaping and learning about healthy boundaries and emotional well-being, I realized much of what I experienced was not normal at all—it was abusive.

Advocating for Systemic Change

While supporting survivors on an individual level is crucial, we must also advocate for systemic change to protect people from emotional and psychological abuse on a broader scale. This includes pushing for stronger legal protections, advocating for mental health support, and addressing the gaps in how society deals with non-physical forms of abuse.

Here are some ways you can advocate for systemic change:

1. **Supporting Legislative Efforts**: Emotional and psychological abuse is often not adequately recognized or addressed in many legal systems. By advocating for laws that expand the definition of domestic abuse to include emotional and psychological harm, we can help ensure that survivors are protected and abusers are held accountable. This might mean advocating for laws that address coercive control, stalking, or other forms of non-physical abuse.

2. **Demanding Mental Health Resources for Survivors**: Emotional abuse can lead to long-term mental health issues such as anxiety, depression, PTSD, Complex-PTSD, and more. Advocating for accessible and affordable mental health care, insurance coverage for therapy, increasing funding for mental health services, and community-based support programs is essential.

3. **Raising Awareness on a National or Global Scale**: Contribute to larger awareness efforts by supporting campaigns that address emotional and psychological abuse. This might mean participating in awareness months (such as Domestic Violence Awareness Month), sharing resources on social media, or even starting your own awareness campaign in your local community.

4. **Collaborating with Advocacy Groups**: Numerous organizations work to prevent emotional abuse and support survivors. By partnering with or supporting these groups, you can help amplify their message and contribute to meaningful change. Some organizations work to raise awareness, while others offer direct services to survivors, such as shelter, counseling, and legal advocacy.

Empowering Yourself and Others to Live Free from Abuse

As we conclude this book, I want to leave you with a message of hope and empowerment. Whether you're a survivor of emotional and psychological abuse, a loved one of someone who has endured it, or an advocate who wants to make a difference, you have the power to create change in your own life and in the lives of others.

Here's how you can continue to empower yourself and others:

1. **Reclaim Your Life**: If you've survived emotional abuse, know that you have the power to reclaim your life. You are not defined by your past or by the abuse you endured. You are strong, resilient, and capable of building a future filled with love, respect, and self-worth. Take the time to heal, to rebuild your confidence, and to pursue the things that bring you joy and fulfillment.

2. **Build Healthy Relationships**: Whether you're a survivor or not, building healthy relationships is essential for personal growth and well-being. Healthy relationships are built on mutual respect, trust, and communication. Surround yourself with people who uplift you, who respect your boundaries, and who celebrate your successes.

3. **Continue Learning and Growing**: The journey of healing and personal growth doesn't end after leaving an abusive relationship—it's a lifelong process. Continue learning about yourself, your needs, and your boundaries. Practice self-awareness and emotional intelligence in all of your relationships, and don't be afraid to seek help or support when you need it.

4. **Support Others on Their Journey**: As you move forward, remember that you have the power to help others on their journey as well. Whether through listening, sharing your story, or advocating for systemic change, you can make a difference in the lives of

survivors and help create a world where emotional and psychological abuse is no longer tolerated.

A Collective Call to Action

Emotional and psychological abuse is a pervasive issue, but it doesn't have to continue unchecked. By recognizing the signs, supporting survivors, and advocating for change, we can create a world where everyone is treated with dignity, respect, and love. This book is just the beginning—the real work happens when we take what we've learned and use it to make a difference.

Together, we can break the silence. Together, we can create a future where emotional abuse is no longer hidden in the shadows. And together, we can empower ourselves and others to live free from manipulation, control, and fear.

Let this be our collective call to action.

APPENDIX

RESOURCES FOR EMOTIONAL ABUSE VICTIMS AND THEIR LOVED ONES

For readers who may find themselves in similar situations or know someone who is, I've compiled a list of resources that can provide support, guidance, and practical help. It's important to recognize the signs of coercive control and understand that emotional and psychological abuse often goes unnoticed but is just as damaging as physical violence.

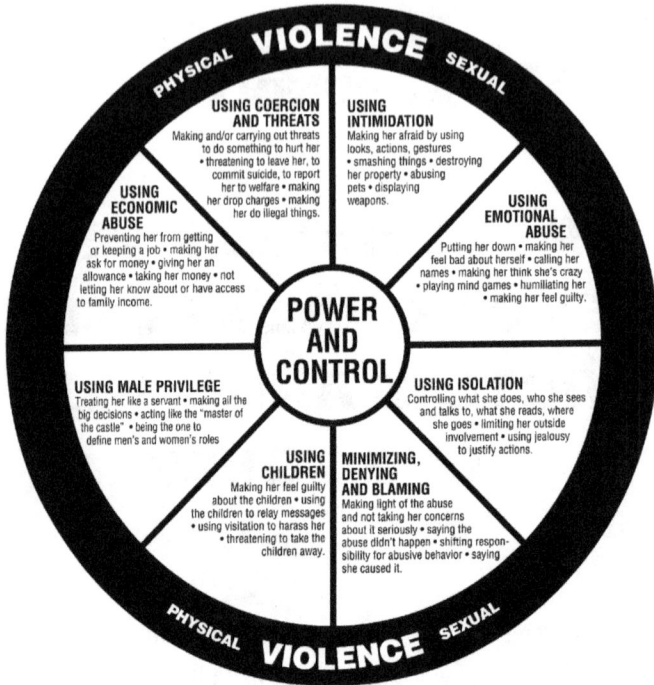

DOMESTIC ABUSE INTERVENTION PROGRAMS
202 East Superior Street
Duluth, Minnesota 55802
218-722-2781
www.theduluthmodel.org

1. Quick Reference Guide: Red Flags of Emotional and Psychological Abuse

Use this quick reference guide to identify red flags and patterns that may indicate emotional abuse. These signs may appear in romantic relationships, friendships, family relationships, or even workplace dynamics.

Early Warning Signs of Emotional and Psychological Abuse:

- **Love Bombing**: Overwhelming attention, compliments, and gifts early in the relationship to create emotional dependence.
- **Excessive Jealousy or Possessiveness**: Displays of jealousy that go beyond normal concern, often resulting in controlling behaviors.
- **Isolation**: Encouraging or demanding that you distance yourself from friends, family, or social activities, making you more dependent on the abuser.
- **Constant Criticism**: Harshly judging your appearance, intelligence, abilities, or decisions, often disguised as "jokes."
- **Gaslighting**: Manipulating you to question your own memory, reality, or perceptions, often making you feel like you're "crazy" or "overreacting."
- **Blaming and Shaming**: Constantly blaming you for the problems in the relationship, making you feel like you're never good enough.
- **Control Over Your Time**: Monitoring where you go, who you see, or what you do, often under the guise of being "protective" or "concerned."

- **Financial Control**: Restricting your access to money, making you dependent on them for basic needs or financial stability.
- **Sudden Mood Swings**: Drastic shifts in their mood or behavior, from loving and attentive one minute to angry and cold the next, keeping you on edge.
- **Threats of Self-Harm or Harm to Others**: Using threats of self-harm or harm to loved ones to keep you from leaving or asserting your independence.
- **Excessive Monitoring of Communications**: Regularly checking your messages, social media, or emails, often claiming it's for your safety.
- **Dictating Personal Choices**: Enforcing strict rules about what you wear, how you act, or who you interact with, further diminishing your autonomy.

Recognizing these signs is the first step in seeking help and regaining control over your life. If you or someone you know is experiencing these forms of abuse, reaching out for support can be a crucial step toward healing.

2. How to Respond to Emotional Abuse

If you suspect that you or someone you love is in an emotionally abusive relationship, it's important to take action. Here's a quick reference guide on how to respond:

If You're Experiencing Emotional Abuse:

- **Acknowledge the Abuse**: Recognize that emotional abuse is real, and you deserve to be treated with respect, love, and kindness.
- **Talk to Someone You Trust**: Reach out to a close friend, family member, or therapist who can offer support and validate your feelings.
- **Document the Abuse**: Keep a record of incidents, behaviors, or patterns of emotional abuse. This can be useful if you need to seek legal or professional help later on.
- **Seek Professional Help**: Consider talking to a therapist or counselor who specializes in emotional abuse and trauma. They can help you navigate your emotions and plan a way forward.
- **Create a Safety Plan**: If the abuse escalates or becomes dangerous, create a plan to leave safely. This may involve finding a place to stay, gathering important documents, and having a support system in place.

If You Suspect a Loved One Is Being Emotionally Abused:

- **Listen Without Judgment**: Offer a safe, non-judgmental space for your loved one to talk. Avoid telling them what to do or pressuring them to leave.
- **Validate Their Feelings**: Let them know that their feelings are real and that they don't deserve the abuse.

Reinforce that emotional abuse is just as serious as physical abuse.

- **Offer Practical Help**: Assist them in finding resources, such as support groups, shelters, or therapists. Offer to help with practical tasks, like transportation or finding legal aid.
- **Respect Their Choices**: Leaving an abusive relationship is difficult and often takes time. Support your loved one's decisions, even if they're not ready to leave just yet.
- **Encourage Self-Care**: Emotional abuse can take a toll on mental and physical health. Encourage your loved one to prioritize their well-being and seek professional help if needed.

3. Resources for Victims of Emotional and Psychological Abuse

Here is a list of resources that offer support for victims of emotional and psychological abuse, including hotlines, online communities, and organizations that provide counseling, legal assistance, and emergency services.

National and International Hotlines:

- **National Domestic Violence Hotline (U.S.)**
  Phone: 1-800-799-SAFE (7233)

Website: www.thehotline.org
Available 24/7 for confidential support, resources, and safety planning.

- **Love Is Respect (U.S.)**
  Phone: 1-866-331-9474
  Text: LOVEIS to 22522
  Website: www.loveisrespect.org
  Offers support for young adults and teens in abusive relationships.

- **National Network to End Domestic Violence (U.S.)**
  Website: www.nnedv.org
  Provides resources and tools for survivors, including legal assistance and emergency housing.

- **Women's Aid (U.K.)**
  Phone: 0808 2000 247 (24-hour helpline)
  Website: www.womensaid.org.uk
  Offers support for women experiencing domestic violence, including emotional abuse.

- **National Center for Domestic and Sexual Violence (U.S.)**
  Website: www.ncdsv.org
  Provides resources and advocacy for survivors of domestic violence and emotional abuse.

- **Rape, Abuse & Incest National Network (RAINN) (U.S.)**
  Phone: 1-800-656-HOPE (4673)
  Website: www.rainn.org

Offers confidential support for survivors of sexual abuse and domestic violence, including emotional abuse.

- **Domestic Violence Resource Centre Victoria (Australia)**
  Website: www.dvrcv.org.au
  Provides resources, support, and education for those experiencing domestic violence, including emotional abuse.

4. Online Communities and Support Groups

Support Groups for Emotional Abuse Survivors:

- **DomesticShelters.org**
  Website: www.domesticshelters.org
  Offers an extensive directory of local shelters, as well as articles and resources for survivors of emotional abuse. Their site also provides a way to connect with online support groups.
- **Out of the Fog**
  Website: www.outofthefog.website
  Offers support for people dealing with emotional abuse and manipulation, especially in relationships with personality disorders (narcissism, borderline, etc.).

- **Reddit – r/abusiverelationships**
  Website: www.reddit.com/r/abusiverelationships
  A supportive community for individuals who are or
  have been in emotionally abusive relationships. Members share advice, personal stories, and resources.
- **Survivors of Emotional Abuse (Facebook Group)**
  Search for "Survivors of Emotional Abuse" on Facebook to join a private support group where members
  can share their stories, offer advice, and support
  one another.
- **IgniteHer** - www.igniteher.org Organization to help
  in the discussion of safe-exit strategies, support and
  education and resource connection.

5. Legal Resources and Advocacy Organizations

If you or a loved one are dealing with the legal aspects of emotional abuse, such as seeking protection orders or custody rights,
these organizations can provide assistance:

Legal Aid and Advocacy:

- **National Coalition Against Domestic Vio-
  lence (NCADV)**
  Website: www.ncadv.org
  Provides resources, legal advocacy, and policy change

initiatives for victims of domestic violence, including emotional and psychological abuse.

- **Legal Aid Society (U.S.)**
  Website: www.legalaid.org
  Offers free legal assistance for survivors of domestic violence, including emotional abuse. Services include help with protection orders, custody, and divorce.
- **Victim Support (U.K.)**
  Website: www.victimsupport.org.uk
  Offers emotional and practical support for victims of crime, including those who have experienced domestic abuse.
- **Break the Silence Against Domestic Violence (U.S.)**
  Website: www.breakthesilencedv.org
  Provides support, advocacy, and resources for survivors of domestic violence, with a focus on emotional and psychological abuse.

6. Self-Care and Healing Resources

Healing from emotional and psychological abuse is a long and complex journey. The following resources offer tools for self-care, mental health support, and personal empowerment:

Books and Reading Materials:

- **The Body Keeps the Score** by Bessel van der Kolk
  A comprehensive guide to understanding how trauma affects the body and mind, with practical tools for healing.
- **Why Does He Do That? Inside the Minds of Angry and Controlling Men** by Lundy Bancroft
  A powerful book that explores the psychology behind abusive behavior and how to break free.
- **Codependent No More** by Melody Beattie
  A book for people in relationships with controlling or manipulative partners, offering strategies for reclaiming independence and self-worth.
- **Is it My Fault? Hope and Healing for Those Suffering** by Lindsey A. Holcomb and Justin S. Holcomb
  A message of hope and healing to victims who know too well the depths of destruction and the overwhelming reality of domestic violence.
- **Dangerous Personalities** by Joe Navarro
  An insightful exploration of various dangerous personality types, helping readers identify red flags in relationships.
- **Why Don't We Ask Why** by Dr. Janina Fisher
  A compelling examination of the complexities of trauma and the importance of asking difficult questions for healing.

Self-Care Apps and Tools:

- **Calm (App)**
  A mindfulness app that offers guided meditations, sleep stories, and tools for stress management. Available on iOS and Android.
- **Sanvello (App)**
  An app designed to help users manage anxiety, depression, and PTSD through cognitive-behavioral therapy (CBT) techniques. Available on iOS and Android.
- **Talkspace (App)**
  An online therapy platform that connects users with licensed therapists for virtual counseling sessions. Available on iOS and Android.

Emotional and psychological abuse is often hidden, but with the right resources and support, survivors can heal, rebuild their lives, and regain their self-worth. This appendix offers just a starting point for those in need of help, as well as for loved ones who want to support someone they care about. Remember, you are not alone—there are people and organizations ready to help.

If you or someone you know is experiencing emotional abuse, don't hesitate to reach out for help. Whether through a hotline, a support group, or a trusted friend, the first step toward healing is speaking out and seeking support.

7. Checklist

It's important to recognize that abuse can take many forms, and even a few signs may indicate an unhealthy or dangerous relationship. If any items on this list feel familiar, trust your instincts. Remember, you are not alone, and there is help available to support your safety and well-being.

Domestic Abuse Self-Assessment Checklist

Physical and Intimidation Tactics

- ☐ Physical harm (hitting, slapping, choking, pushing, etc.)
- ☐ Threats to harm you, loved ones, pets, or themselves
- ☐ Destruction of belongings or home to intimidate
- ☐ Uses weapons or implies threats with weapons

Emotional and Psychological Control

- ☐ Isolates you from friends, family, or social activities
- ☐ Shows extreme jealousy over time spent with others
- ☐ Constantly criticizes or belittles you, especially in public
- ☐ Gaslights (makes you question your perception or reality)

- ☐ Controls your decision-making (e.g., job, school)
- ☐ Shifts blame, making you feel responsible for their behavior
- ☐ Alternates between extreme affection and sudden coldness
- ☐ Uses silent treatment or withdrawal as punishment
- ☐ Has unpredictable mood swings, causing fear of "triggering" them

Financial Control

- ☐ Restricts access to money or controls all household finances
- ☐ Forces financial dependency by preventing employment or promotions
- ☐ Spends or takes money without consent

Sexual and Coercive Behavior

- ☐ Pressures or forces you into unwanted sexual activity
- ☐ Controls your sexual or reproductive decisions
- ☐ Threatens self-harm or suicide if you don't comply
- ☐ Threatens to expose personal information or make false accusations

Digital and Social Media Abuse

- ☐ Monitors your devices, messages, or social media without consent, or with forced consent
- ☐ Sends threatening or harassing messages, posting embarrassing content
- ☐ Threatens to publicly share personal information
- ☐ Uses digital tools to track your location or movements

Social Manipulation

- ☐ Publicly shames, humiliates, or belittles you
- ☐ Sabotages your goals (work, school, personal aspirations)
- ☐ Uses third parties to control or intimidate you (triangulation)

For Friends and Family Observing Potential Abuse

- ☐ They isolate from family and friends, withdrawing from social circles
- ☐ Shows sudden changes in behavior, becoming fearful, jumpy or anxious
- ☐ Has unexplained injuries or frequently covers up parts of their body
- ☐ Expresses new financial stress or restriction from their partner

- ☐ Appears insecure, disempowered or overly deferential around their partner

If you think you may be in an abusive relationship, consider developing a personal safety plan that includes steps like identifying safe people to contact, gathering essentials (IDs, money), and practicing ways to exit quickly. Reach out to a trusted friend, family member, or professional. You can also contact The National Domestic Violence Hotline at 800.799.SAFE (7233) for confidential support. Remember, leaving an abusive relationship can be complex and may require planning for your safety. Seek assistance to ensure you have the resources and support you need.